MENDING REALITY

AN ADVOCATE'S EXISTENTIAL JOURNEY WITH MENTAL HEALTH

COHEN MILES-RATH

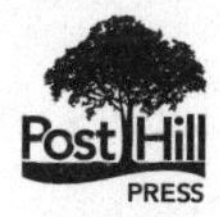

A POST HILL PRESS BOOK
ISBN: 979-8-89565-002-8
ISBN (eBook): 979-8-89565-003-5

Mending Reality:
An Advocate's Existential Journey with Mental Health

Cover design by Cody Corcoran
Cover photo by Delconte Photography LLC

All people, locations, events, and situations are portrayed to the best of the author's memory. While all of the events described are true, many names and identifying details have been changed to protect the privacy of the people involved.

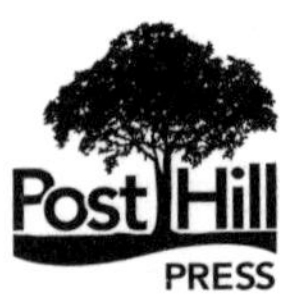

Post Hill Press
New York • Nashville
posthillpress.com

Published in the United States of America
1 2 3 4 5 6 7 8 9 10

Advance Praise for *Mending Reality*

"Miles-Rath's account of his 2016 onset of schizoaffective disorder at the age of twenty-two is a must-read. He communicates the experience of psychosis with the clarity and humanity that only someone with lived experience can. Just as importantly, Miles-Rath highlights the ways that even the best-intentioned policies fail the millions who experience psychosis, particularly the small percentage whose delusions lead to violence. His story reveals how our mental health system struggles at every level—from early intervention to crisis response to recovery support. We must amplify voices like Miles-Rath's to correct damaging narratives about mental illness that promote stigma, enable ineffective and dehumanizing treatment, deny dignity and autonomy, and fail to support meaningful recovery. This memoir stands as both a gripping personal account and an urgent call for systemic change. Well-written, relatable, and highly recommended."

—Sophie Littlefield, author and
mental health advocate

for my father

CONTENTS

PART IV

AUTHOR'S NOTE

Everything in this book is from my memory, a collection of records, research, and conversations with family and friends. I don't remember everything from my experience with psychosis—this story is a small fraction. I know some memories were severe delusions, hallucinations, and other symptoms. With other memories, I don't know if they were a symptom or not. I want to keep it that way. If I were to summarize coping with my psychosis, it would be the ability to acknowledge and embrace the gap between certainty and uncertainty.

For explanation ease, I use well-known clinical terms to describe my experience with mental illness. I understand these experiences could be described differently and apart from the medical model. I value these perspectives and support the growing conversation with mental health.

The majority of people's names in this book are pseudonyms.

Content Warning

Many parts of this book may be difficult for those who have experienced psychosis or psychosis-related symptoms. Please read with caution and do not continue if symptoms occur. Also included are depictions of mania, suicide, self-harm, and violence. Please reach out to a trusted source if you need help. For immediate support, call or text 988 or chat at 988lifeline.org.

FOREWORD

Two months after I published my memoir, a man named Cohen sent me a message on Facebook.

"We have a similar story," he began, "although I was the one holding the knife."

The book I had just published was about this similar story. More than a decade before I spoke with Cohen, my younger brother, Tim, began struggling with schizophrenia. Years of attempted treatment and hospitalization did little to quiet his mounting illness. In 2014, in the midst of a severe psychosis, Tim attacked and killed our mother.

One of the differences between Cohen's story and my own is that his father survived.

"My father was able to fight me off," Cohen's message explained, "avoiding a life ending tragedy for my family."

But Cohen and Tim shared many things. They shared a diagnosis, a winding path of inadequate treatment, obstacles preventing them from receiving the care they needed. They had both been serious college athletes. Both had studied philosophy. They were both twenty-two when psychosis convinced them that one of their parents needed to die.

Cohen's life, of course, diverged dramatically from Tim's. After thirty days in jail and a year of mandatory treatment, Cohen went on to earn a master's degree in social work, start a career as a mental health advocate, tell his story to enact needed change. Tim has been confined in a psychiatric prison for over a decade.

When I agreed to speak with Cohen, I told him that I was captivated by his story and in awe of his work as an advocate. This was—and remains—true. But there was something else, something I couldn't say or explain to him at the time. I needed to speak with Cohen, so I could see who Tim might have become if our mother had survived.

Among the many powerful currents running through Cohen's book is a haunting string of *what if.* Cohen injects these moments into his gripping narrative, pausing the scenes in which his illness seizes control to wonder how else his story could have unfolded. The sharpest is the one that animates the book, the *what if* at his story's core.

Imagine where I would be now if that knife punctured my father's throat. He wouldn't be here. I'd be locked up somewhere. Psychosis still tormenting me.

Many moments in Cohen's narrative receive this treatment. He rigorously interrogates his past.

What if I went through a less frightening method of urgent care—would have I been more likely to listen to the doctors? What if, instead of forced medication, treatment relied on support from loved ones, peers, and providers who engaged in a process of change rather than an immediate fix?

What if I understood what schizophrenia was—would I have taken it more seriously?

Though all of us can understand the impulse behind these questions—did this have to happen, what could have changed—those of us with intimate knowledge of mental illness—whether firsthand or through a loved one—know how what if, what if, what if can spiral out of control. I have plenty what ifs of my own.

What if I had listened to Tim when he told me he saw a possessed coin floating in our basement? What if Tim had taken his pills instead of flushing them down the toilet? What if our mother had dialed 911 before he attacked her? What if I had been at home on the day our mother died?

Sometimes, guilt animates what if. For a long time, guilt was behind most of mine.

But Cohen's what ifs are the basis for investigation, for digging into his past for something more profound than why, why, why. His book points a way forward, conceives of a world where we recognize the early signs of mental illness, where we eliminate barriers to effective treatment, where we pay attention when someone is in the grip of psychosis.

In describing what being in this grip meant for him, Cohen offers the most piercing first-hand account of psychosis that I have ever read. This includes everything from sensory disruptions ("The red paint's glossy texture smoldered against the night's shadow,") to bizarre acts stemming from delusions ("To show the devil I could get rid of him, I smashed a building's window and tossed in red items including a hat, lighter, and an Old Spice container,") to world mangling messages ("His black clothes. His red face.... The devil is inside my dad,").

But what these details provide, in addition to riveting narrative, is an antidote to all the sensationalized headlines that flattened Cohen's story after he attacked his father. As he points out, those articles about the attack remain one Google search away, the single column stories that cast him in the stigmatized role of deranged killer.

I can't stop people from searching for my name. I could change it—John Michael is common enough to remove me from the spotlight. But I need my identity.

And we need it too: the Cohen in this book, the full picture he provides of childhood, madness, and recovery. So much more than a mug shot in a newspaper.

This is also what I needed for Tim. In the aftermath of our mother's death, the word *Matricide* appeared in sensationalized headlines, invoking horror films that condition us to see Tim as the psycho killer of our nightmares.

It has always been easier for us to treat people like Cohen and Tim as monsters. It's easier to dismiss their stories with a single headline, with the specter of the deranged killer. It's easier to scoff "psycho" and cast their stories aside.

But Cohen's book suggests another way. What if we saw the full story behind these headlines? What if we understood how serious mental illnesses can metastasize in the people we love? What if we paid attention instead of looking away?

At first, I did see Cohen as a version of my brother, as who Tim could have become on a more hopeful timeline, one where our mother didn't have to die. How could I not have? Yet, as I got to know Cohen, as I read his writing, another painful wish emerged. What if I had met Cohen before my mother died?

If I'd heard Cohen's story or read this book—then, before—I would have known how corrosive Tim's demons could become. I would have known about the barriers to effective treatment for people living with psychosis. I would have known that at the apex of Tim's untreated illness our mother's life could be in danger.

In the opening of this book, Cohen wonders, "What small mercy kept my family and me from plunging into this darkness?" Of course, this question is painful for me. The small mercy that saved Cohen's father was absent when my mother died.

But with *Mending Reality*, Cohen has given us more than a small mercy. He's written something that will inspire systemic change and save lives. He's crafted a story for people facing challenges with their mental health and a story that will make a difference for families on the precipice of crisis.

I know it could have made a difference for mine.

Vince Granata, author of *Everything Is Fine*
October 2024

PART I

PRISONER

Trapped in a jail cell, I sit on its wall-anchored table. Rotting flesh—cuisine from Hell's Kitchen—feeds my nostrils. I haven't eaten in days.

I stare at the wall—its white, dirty cement. Little dots are wedged within the concrete like scattered stars in the dark.

I'm seeing the Universe. It's disintegrating. Dripping. Dropping. The dots fade right before me.

"He…lp," a static voice pleads through the radio—the only way for cross-galaxy contact.

It's all my fault. I discovered the key to existence. I let it slip into Satan's grip.

But wait. I can stop this. I control everything. Maybe, I can connect the dots and fix everything.

I strengthen my focus. My back straightens. My head steadies. I feel the air lift—the dots stay afloat. It's working.

"You got this. Our world cheers for you!" another voice from beyond the horizon says.

I'm fixating so intensely, I shake. Biceps bounce. Shoulders convulse.

"Stop playing games!" shouts the Man in Black from outside the cell door.

My focus veers. I lose my grip. Pressure pounds on my brain as the cheers grow louder, and the wall flashes like a vicious strobe light.

All I can think is how I am so close. So close to finishing the mission.

But the pressure pounds on my brain; the pressure pounds on my brain; the pressure pounds on my brain.

I stop, right before the Universe mends. Screaming cuts the air. Sounds of terror from those who cheered me on.

Guilt. Shame. I feel a presence.

"Where is he?" a sinister voice asks the Man in Black.

I look down. My arms shine bright red. The white floor blurs my periphery.

"I'm going to talk to Satan."

"Don't talk to Satan."

Heavy foul footsteps approach my cell.

"Hey, Brother."

I look around, dazed.

"Go to bed and stop playing games," the prison guard says.

I listen.

I stood tall when reading this poem—two years since that jail cell—in front of strangers. Mouths dropped. Eyes stretched wide. Clearly, not everyone in the audience had heard a first-hand experience of severe psychosis.

Hallucinations of Satan and Gods. Delusions of discovering the truth in everything. A deceptive connection to the Universe.

I didn't mention how I ended up in jail. I tried to kill my dad because I believed the devil was inside him. I wasn't ready to talk about that yet.

Others went on to read their poems—happy, soft words that brought light into the room.

"It's a great day for poetry," one reader said.

I agreed—it was my first time.

People circled me after the event.

"Thank you so much for sharing," an older woman said, grabbing my hand and tilting her eyes up.

"Not everyone appreciates the dark poet," a middle-aged man said. "They always want the merry ones."

Then an older man, with one hand on my shoulder and the other cupping his mouth, leaned into my ear.

"I suffer from depression and had suicidal thoughts not that long ago," he whispered, as if saying something bad. "Thank you for sharing."

His somber voice warmed my heart. I wasn't the only one looking for support.

* * *

I wrote the poem in my bedroom during graduate school. A room the same size as that jail cell from two years before. Both fit a twin-size bed, desk, and little walking room. However, in the bedroom, my state of reality was far different.

I had freedom. I could open a window and smell the fresh air of nearby trees. I could decorate with my favorite images—pictures of friends, a New York City poster, and art depicting the Adirondack Mountains.

I had mental stability. Nothing forced me to believe in anything out of the ordinary. I knew the exact time and day, and could understand what I was doing. Most importantly, I knew who I was.

I was Cohen. A young man, born and raised in rural New York, pursuing a master's degree in social work to help others. Although my mind, body, and soul were no longer bound by the shackles that once pulled me into the dark abyss, I didn't live without them.

* * *

If you Google my name right now, you find news articles from the spring of 2016, the year I was to graduate from college. One is titled "Steuben County Man Accused of Assaulting Father."

If you read that article, you learn how I attacked my dad with a knife. I bit a chunk of his ear off. Police arrested me at gunpoint. As my dad went to the hospital, I went to jail. Both of us were terrified of the future.

What you don't learn, however, is that I was facing a mental health crisis. You don't learn what could have been done to prevent the incident. You don't learn that it was a miracle for my dad and me to survive. Only his thumb had blocked the blade's tip from puncturing his throat. Millimeters that separated his life from death—and mine from the torment of killing someone I loved so much.

These articles, still floating around the internet's ether, have tormented me. How would employers feel if they found out? What about girls on first dates or future roommates?

I can't stop people from searching for my name. I could change it—John Michael is common enough to remove me from the spotlight. But I need my identity.

I can't change who I am; psychosis did enough of that.

So what can I do?

Understand my mental health. Examine what we can address on the individual, community, and systemic level. Share my story to advocate for change.

I've accepted what happened. I've rebuilt my life. I now embrace those articles, using everything I have learned to support my mission of improving our mental health approach.

Seven years after that jail cell, I spoke to a crowd of over two hundred at Mental Health Matters Day, joining advocates at the New York State Capitol.

"When I think of mental health advocacy, I think about how impactful this work is. Without it, I might not be here today," I said, before sharing my story.

Mouths dropped again. Clearly, we need to hear more first-hand experiences of psychosis.

We need to prevent crises such as mine.

* * *

The more I learn about mental health, the more I understand how my mind fell ill and distorted my life. For many, mental illness varies, and its impact ranges. Had my situation gone slightly differently, I'd still be suffering in prison.

What small mercy kept my family and me from plunging into this darkness?

What separates me from Timothy Granata? A young man who experienced untreated schizophrenia and killed his mom before graduating college in 2014. Someone who has spent years in an institution more like a jail than a mental health support community.

What about Zack McDermott? A twenty-six-year-old man whose untreated bipolar led him to think his life was a movie. Through a manic episode with psychosis in 2009, he believed he was receiving messages from the TV. His erratic behavior on Manhattan streets resulted in his arrest on a subway platform.

Or Daniel Prude from Rochester, New York—sixty miles from where I grew up. In 2020, Daniel faced a mental health crisis in which he walked the city streets naked. When his family called for help, police killed Daniel with a spit hood.

These situations are painful and terrifying, and they strengthen my resolve to advocate for change. Because the more our mental health approach improves, the more likely we can build a supportive community and reduce people's suffering.

I hope my journey illustrates a person's struggle, recovery, and the need to prioritize mental health. However, this is more than a story of mental illness.

This is a story of seeking the ultimate truth of reality—a mission I believed had been granted to me by the Universe—and how I derived a sentence to save the world. But instead, it bled my mind and troubled my spirit into oblivion.

I'm still finding my way back.

SPLIT START

I never knew what life was like as a baby—how my parents would pinch my chubby cheeks or change my diaper. I never knew what I felt when the sun first brightened my soft, pale skin. Life was a mystery. A mystery pieced together by the world around me.

Eventually, others told me how my life began on November 21, 1993, and filled the gaps of my early years. I saw old faded photographs of my wide eyes and blue baseball shirt. As I grew, I believed everything I was told.

A belief in what others say.

One of my earliest memories is with my dad. I was five. In the living room of his home, I sat scrunched up in his arms, crying and pleading for my mom not to take me. I looked into her cautious eyes, screaming bloody murder as she pulled me away.

I told my parents about this memory years later. My dad recalled me slapping her, adding how satisfied he felt. My little body on his chest, rejecting the other half, signaled to him that she was wrong for taking me. My mom, on the other hand, doesn't remember and questioned if it ever happened.

The subjectivity of memory.

* * *

I never knew much about my parent's separation. I heard a different story when in conversation, whether with them or a sibling. Pieces of a puzzle that, if put together, would portray an abstract mirage—a representation of the miscommunication seemingly bound to my family's history. No matter the uncertainty, the tone was ugly.

My half-sister Karmen, who my mom birthed at eighteen, told me how she took my siblings and me to a motel after the separation. Being six years older, she could remember. We then moved in with Mom's new boyfriend and his two children.

The house was gray with red trim—a novel look. Down the street from my dad's, I could walk to his place in one minute. However, I could only make the walk when the court said so. I had become a pawn in the custody battle between my parents.

Like children fighting over a toy, both tried to get what they wanted. I heard many accusations throughout the years.

Disagreements. Money issues. Mom said this. Dad said that. *Blah blah blah.*

Ultimately for me, it was he-said, she-said bullshit and a dreadful time for a boy whose life was just beginning. A boy whose wish for his parents to reunite never came true.

* * *

After my mom won primary custodianship, she married her boyfriend—a wedding I didn't attend because my dad didn't want me to. Then the assorted group of step, half-, and full-blooded relatives moved fifteen miles from my dad.

In the rural town of Dansville, New York, our new house had shabby carpets and dingy furniture. Its wallpaper turned yellow due to years of cigarette smoke.

The three girls shared a bedroom while the three boys shared another. With one shower, reusing bath water sufficed sometimes.

Family-cooked meals were uncommon. Instead, kids ate food from a can or box—mostly afforded by food stamps.

We had to ask for items from the fridge. Milk. Eggs. Leftover pizza. But we always looked forward to our special treat—McDonald's chicken nuggets, McFlurries, and Happy Meal toys.

My mom was a school lunch lady and nurse and worked hard to provide. She once bought me the new Spiderman video game—sixty dollars she struggled to afford. I would wake up before anyone else to play. She'd sit beside me and watch.

My mom would say that my dad favored me over my half-siblings. Oftentimes, it felt like she and my stepdad showed favoritism to their biological children as well.

I was close with Casie, my stepsister of the same age. When I felt my mom treated her unfairly, I'd get back at her by wiping sticky boogers on her bedroom door knob.

I didn't know what my stepdad did for work. One time, the wrong child ate his eggs. He spun his truck in the driveway, spitting pebbles at the house. We kids ducked beneath the sill as windows popped and cracked. Our breakfast suddenly felt like a war zone.

Divided families. Squabbles for control. Who paid for whose clothes? Who sets the rules?

Power struggles fractured the house. Without discretionary income, raising six children was demanding.

* * *

My siblings and I took advantage of the dysfunction. Lindsay, the second-oldest half-sister, and Karmen would often babysit. They used board games such as Monopoly to keep us close. However, they struggled to manage the four of us closer in age: Cody, my half-brother, Taylor, my stepbrother, Casie, and myself.

Being outside was our go-to. The quiet countryside allowed us to play on the streets without fearing cars. We held races on bikes. We investigated abandoned buildings. We rolled dried leaves and smoked them like cigarettes.

Cody would challenge my skateboarding skills. I was terrified of the quarter pipe.

"C'mon, little bro," he'd say. "I got you."

Taylor invented a game called Death Part City. Dressed in battle gear of garbage can tops and blanket capes, we traveled to other dimensions, fighting evil spirits.

"I dub Cohen, the knight of this city. Together, we will save the world," he said, handing me a stick sword.

Anything could be a portal—a hula hoop, a hole in the fence, a gap in the tree where I once fell due to the collapse of my brothers' treehouse. As the youngest, I was the test dummy.

Inside the home, we stayed up wrestling, not caring if a head smashed a hole in the wall. My mom and stepdad would call us downstairs at one in the morning to squish our bodies in a corner. We'd smirk at each other.

Tee hee tee haha haha. Crescendoing giggles mocked our punishment.

Some of our expeditions bridged the law. One night, we explored the Girl Scout Park after hours. When a police officer's spotlight appeared, we darted into bushes—more thrill than fear.

Another time, a store attendant caught Taylor stealing a candy bar. A picture of his face plastered behind the cash register with the words "Do not let in" was easy for us to laugh at.

We were a proud band of misfits.

* * *

Compared to my siblings, I was less likely to engage in mischief, often referred to as a good child of the family. My relationship with my dad influenced my behavior. Through the custody agreement, I visited him every other weekend and one day each week.

I wanted to be just like my dad. I pierced my ear like him. I copied his leather jacket, boot-wearing blue jeans, and—business in the front, party in the back—mullet. I was a mini-version of an '80s hair band rocker.

My dad, an average-height and stocky man, delivered gas and oil for Griffith Energy Services. He owned a house—a well-kept double-wide trailer—in Cohocton, NY, a one-stoplight town. Aside from a small deli, there was nowhere to eat a meal.

A typical visit to his home included an activity. We traveled to places near and far, once driving hours for a Philly cheesesteak because it was on the Food Channel. We crafted a red-striped wooden car in the Boy Scouts to win the Pinewood Derby Championship. We spent one summer assembling a three-story treehouse that never collapsed underneath me.

Haunted houses became a yearly tradition. I cried the first time I went. The bloody face of an evil clown petrified my little mind. But my dad encouraged me to keep going, sometimes bringing the fright home.

At night, I'd be sitting in our living room when he would disappear. My legs would shake while stepping into the darkened kitchen.

"Daddy, where are you?"

He'd emerge from the pitch-black hallway by my bedroom, making me jump two feet. Over the years, I grew to withstand the fear and enjoy the occasional scare.

It wasn't always fun and games at my dad's. I never wanted to be told to vacuum the couch. I hated cleaning my room and dreaded the springtime when he'd make me stick my knees in the dirt to pull out weeds.

"Be sure not to break off the root," he'd say. "We don't want them growing back."

I listened, though. My dad ensured I had to work for what I wanted, and he would provide. Although he was frugal, comparing produce costs at Walmart and Aldis, for me, he invested.

The second I showed interest in drums, he bought me a set. If I wanted the new Goosebumps book, he'd get it. Video games, however, had to meet his criteria.

Resident Evil qualified. *Tony Hawk's Pro Skater* qualified. But *Grand Theft Auto*—a game where human characters could casually kill each other—I could only play at my mom's.

* * *

Visits to my dad often ended with a homemade meal. He would plop in his recliner with food and a remote in one hand. I'd follow suit.

We would tune into the news hour before flipping on *Touched by an Angel* or *Walker, Texas Ranger*. Their religious undertones taught me some Christian values until 10 p.m. before then lights out.

My mom, although raised Catholic, was agnostic.

"I'm not going to stress about going to Heaven or Hell," she'd say. "You don't need to believe in God to be a good person. You should treat people the way you want to be treated."

With my mom, we never went to church. With my dad, Sundays at church became routine. But we stopped going after a few years. Although my dad identified as Christian, the church wasn't as crucial as its principles.

His standard was evident at one church. I left the main hall for a pee break. When I returned, the doors were locked. They wouldn't let me back in.

"We can't have any disruptions during Mass," staff said.

"He's a kid," my dad argued. "Your doors are always supposed to be open."

We never returned.

"Hypocrites," my dad would say.

I was fine not going. I didn't connect to Jesus or the Holy Bible. I liked the show *VeggieTales* though. Its straightforward optimism to overcome any challenge resonated with me.

I was the sole child at my dad's—a more quiet and reserved person. I had my own room and toys and no need to share anything with anyone.

My sibling's other parents couldn't provide for them in the same way, particularly for my half-siblings. Cody's dad struggled with drugs and passed away in high school from diabetes. Karmen and Lindsay's dad started a new life.

I was often the only one with an expensive gift or Disney World story. As the years went on, I was more likely to boast about what I had.

"You haven't played the new *Guitar Hero* yet? Too busy smoking weed?" was something I would have said to my siblings.

Like the church, I was a hypocrite too. As I got older, I'd light up any chance I could get.

* * *

I never felt the need to know the truth as to why my parents split. I could not grasp their conflict when I was young, and as I grew, I realized they had separate lives. Separate lives that wanted to be involved in mine.

Grateful.

My mom had her challenges. As a child, she moved throughout the country—split parents fighting over her and her brother. The family struggled to ground its roots and create opportunity. But with me and my siblings, she found her home. I never doubted her love for us.

I told my mom I wanted to live with my dad often. One day, she saw me hiding tears.

"What's wrong?" she asked, holding my hands.

"I want to live with my dad."

I sensed her feeling defeated. No loving mom would want to hear their child's rejection. But no loving dad would want to miss the opportunity to raise their child. Most importantly, no kid would want to choose between loving parents.

Yet there I was less than ten years of age, making that decision. Eventually, I knew what I wanted and advocated for it.

Before sixth grade, my mom removed her custodianship, allowing me to live with my dad. I agreed to visit her house every other weekend and one day each week. I wanted to see her and my siblings. At least I had a voice in the decision this time.

I wasn't the only one to leave my mom's. Taylor and Casie moved to their mom's. Karmen moved in with her high-school boyfriend. Cody and Lindsay lived with our grandpa for a brief time.

Like my mom, my dad had challenges growing up. Although he had a place to call home, the same town he continued to live in, he had minimal opportunities. Lack of money meant he could never pursue his college dreams. Then a family tragedy struck. His chance of a better future increased in difficulty.

Until he had a son.

My dad told me I resembled his younger brother Steven—my middle name. An uncle I never met who passed away from cancer at thirteen.

One night, when I was in my early teens, my dad arrived home really late.

"Where were you?" I asked, afraid for his safety.

"Visiting Stevie's grave," he said. "It's his birthday."

I felt stupid not knowing my uncle's birthday. But my dad rarely talked about his death. When he did, he described how it happened before Christmas. A pile of presents left unopened—a family heartbroken.

I always felt my dad's love was much more profound than giving me what he didn't have as a child. It was more than attention and financial support.

It was guardianship. It was unconditional. It was why he fought for me to live with him.

* * *

Before and after my parent's separation, they recorded home videos. In these tapes, I see us as we were.

I see our first home together. Its tacky carpets and wallpaper, the '80s-style velvet couch. I see my siblings and I opening

Christmas gifts in the living room. We grinned and chuckled—brief moments when we were a whole family.

I see the separation. My dad slow-danced with me—only me—in his arms. Dimness encompassed the windows of that same living room as we swayed back and forth, singing a rock ballad.

"You're so important to me," he'd say.

Alone but together, my dad and I were an inseparable duo.

My mom's videos captured the six kids standing in ordered lines, creating an exuberant dance to a movie scene from *Shrek*. The house shook. Game Boys and Barbie dolls tumbled off their shelves.

One video caught Cody and I jamming to a rock song.

"You gotta jump to the music little bro," he shouted.

Both of us had sufficient hair to achieve pure head-banging quality.

Several videos captured me taking the stage floor. I danced. I sang solo in my Harry Potter and SpongeBob SquarePants jammies. Sometimes, I talked and talked and talked, heaving any word that rang a bell in my mind.

The person I was then was the person I grew up to be. Someone with joy, passion, and an appreciation for those around me. Even when the dark side of life reared its ugly head, I sought hope. Hope for a better life.

My family may have never been traditional or together, but we had each other. I was always thankful for that. Because later, when I suffered, I'd return home and rely on my family.

A journey that began when I found success in a pair of running shoes.

Toeing the line.

* * *

I am the product of the environment in which I grew up. My family. My privileges and disadvantages. How I looked and what I did—cultural and social differences. My hometown.

I know my home wasn't typical, and my parents did their best. I never needed wealth to feel loved, and I'm not ashamed of my childhood.

Through resilience, I've come to terms with my adverse childhood experiences, also known as ACEs. I have learned how they can increase the likelihood of future challenges such as risky behaviors and socioeconomic difficulties.

I'm not alone in this. My mother had ACEs. My father had ACEs. More than half of all adults have experienced at least one ACE. Intergenerational disadvantages can impact so many of us, and I sometimes feel torn considering their ACEs and my own.

After my mental illness, my father described his attempted suicide after Steven's passing. He told me about his bipolar diagnosis—how he didn't care about it. Like the abstract mirage of my family's history, this genetic predisposition stayed quiet and ignored.

Why?

My family didn't talk about mental health. We struggled to open up—to reveal how we felt and listen nonjudgmentally. But what would it have been like if we did?

Alongside ACEs, I frequently shifted my personality to match my home life. Extroversion and rebelliousness at my mother's. Introversion and obedience at my father's. I often felt uncertain about what was right, wrong, and questionable. All children experience differentiation—the critical learning process in child development—but I was presented with an extreme form.

My father gave me more attention and financial benefits. But I now realize his rules and money made me judge my siblings and see them as lesser although I was no different than them.

Would I have been better off if my parents co-parented adequately? What if my father went to college, or my mother's jobs allowed her to provide more support? What if I was born into a family with discretionary income—would I care about the needs of those who are not?

I changed when I moved into my father's house, and now realize how his presence and support helped inspire me to succeed. Though I wasn't sure exactly what "success" might entail, his encouragement of sports allowed me to seize opportunity and take action.

GOING THE DISTANCE

The first time I laced up was in kindergarten. My parents took me to a field day at the school. I was to race one lap around the track.

I didn't win. My only competitor—a girl—kicked my ass. But I didn't care. The quarter mile of youthful energy—no fear, no doubt—was cathartic. So much so that I joined a running club from third to fifth grade.

The club held a mile race every year. I became hard to beat, taking first place multiple times.

"You're cheating," one kid would constantly say.

"Stop lying," I'd say. "I never cheat."

I follow the rules.

I was no saint, however. At some point, I learned that boys should be better than girls. The next time one gapped my stride, I stuck my leg out, and she fell. Tears followed—blood dripping down her leg.

I felt immediate guilt. But I couldn't retract. Pride was taking its toll.

I gained my dad's approval through running. Together, we took my champion certificates, flattened them under a soft wooden frame, and suspended them above family photos in our home. We admired their gold borders and "1st Place" words every day.

"If you work hard, you can be anything you want when you grow up," my dad often told me.

* * *

I didn't know anyone at my new middle school. Initially, I was an outcast, taunted for my mullet.

I let kids take pictures of me, ignoring their snickers. I didn't understand the hate; I loved my mullet. The way it blew in the wind as I ran. How my dad and I styled it every morning, my forehead sticky with hairspray.

Although my siblings were no longer there to be my friends, it didn't take me long to find one. I met Finn on the first day of sixth grade. Straight out of Catholic school with a Tupac T-shirt and bling necklace, he was also a square peg in a round hole.

No one sat with us in history class. But it didn't matter. One day, our teacher assigned a group project. We were to build a Styrofoam model of the Blarney Castle in Ireland.

He was excited about spray paint. I was along for the ride. We met at a trail in the woods when we discovered our homes were within walking distance. Finn wanted to show me some of his work on these cement blocks—remnants of an old building no longer there.

"If Gandhi can, you can," he read, pointing to yellow squiggly lines.

At that moment, I knew how fortunate I was to have a master of spray paint on my team.

Our adventures grew throughout the years. The trail was a go-to place, and many nights we stayed up playing a *Call of Duty* video game or exploring the abandoned cheese factory.

We reenacted battles in my backyard. Finn charged the tree fortress with a BB gun as I shot at him with a branch.

Pew pew. Our pressed lips mimicked bullet shots.

My dad invited Finn on a trip to Gettysburg, Pennsylvania. After a quick stop for Philly cheesesteaks, we honored the battlefields of American history. More vacations followed—a cruise to Mexico and a trip to New York City.

When high school arrived, Finn and I formed a punk rock band called FISM (Five Incredibly Sexy Men). We jammed at local churches and community centers, once winning a Battle of the Bands because half our school showed up. His microphone and my drums instantly made us the cool kids.

Finn became a brother—a friend to grow up with. Even when I picked up the sport of long-distance running, he joined me.

* * *

I wanted to be a part of running as much as possible. I joined cross-county and indoor and outdoor track. My dad and I befriended the families of the team. I was inspired by Olympic runner Steve Prefontaine, attaching his quote, "To give anything less than your best is to sacrifice the gift," to my Facebook profile.

When I turned fourteen—the age my dad allowed me to date—I found a girlfriend through the sport. Luckily for Sarah—a girl with soft brown hair and teal eyes—I changed my appearance to meet teenage fashion standards.

No longer did I have my mullet. Instead, I let my hair grow out. I swapped my leather jacket for a Blink-182 punk rock shirt and skinny jeans. Vans classic slip-ons replaced my boots. I even quit wearing an earring.

'80s rocker to scene kid.

Sarah and I were captivated by each other within months of dating. We made out in the hallways and the school's backwoods. We scheduled our classes together to cross paths during the day. When cell phones came around, texting was a priority.

Soon enough, we talked about spending our life together. At the time, I couldn't see myself with anyone else. Although I followed my dad's age rule with dating, he wasn't okay with the relationship's blooming nature.

One day, I found anti-sex pamphlets on the couch. I tossed them on the ottoman—a few falling onto the floor. It would get worse.

"You can't prevent me from seeing her!" I shouted when he put a cap on our visits. "It's not fair."

"Don't you care about running?" he shouted back. "That should be your focus, not spending all your time with her."

I didn't understand; Sarah greatly supported my running career. But I couldn't change anything. He was the parent.

The tension between my dad and me grew to the point where I ran away. Literally and figuratively, I trekked ten miles to Sarah's front door. However, my futile liberation only granted me a few minutes with her.

"Get home, or I'm calling the police," he'd say on the phone.

What a prick.

* * *

Popularity was new to me. By the time I was a sophomore, I had a girlfriend, I was a drummer, and I became *the runner*. No longer were people snickering at me. They knew me and only took pictures of me for my talents.

I flourished the most with running. I started to win big races, smiling when the school's announcements read my name. "Congrats, Cohen" became a familiar phrase entering my ears and pumping my ego. A moment arrived, however, when I realized running was much more significant than recognition.

On a spring day, I rode with a buddy to a dirt road on the outskirts of town. After our four-mile run, he drove back. I continued. The only way to get home was to trek on roads I'd never run. Something about that uncertainty—that feeling of being lost yet knowing where you're headed—slowed time for me.

Step after step, I lifted each leg off the cemented ground. Hints of pain and pleasure sweat through my skin. I savored the touch of damp wind and floral scents.

Sounds of nature sung with what I saw: cloud-like shapes of rolling hills, gentle and smooth. Grass and leaves bloomed in the new year, rich with green vibrancy.

My thoughts were as clear as can be. Like air soaring through the creases of space and time, I felt weightlessness wash over me.

I wasn't a person with worries or dreams. I wasn't bound by what society made of me or what I thought of myself.

I felt free. I felt present. I felt alive.

Before reaching my house, I turned, adding another loop. Then I ran another. And another. By the time I finished, I must have run a half-marathon. I didn't want it to end.

When I stopped, I sat—a still pause on the front steps. I felt the calm yet intense serenity of pushing myself beyond a limit I had never reached before.

I pondered the next steps in my life.

How far could running take me?

* * *

I met Coach Dan during my freshman year of high school. I was running a solo workout at track practice when he matched my pace. Ten years older—same height and stride—he had been a successful distance runner at SUNY Geneseo.

"I hear you're the fastest runner," he said. "I'm gonna be your assistant coach. Tell me about yourself."

I never understood pure dedication to a sport until Coach Dan arrived. He often referred to the concept of the *twenty-four-hour-seven-days-a-week athlete*. A standard that required a strict sleep routine, exercise, healthy habits, and consideration of how each moment affected running.

I put hours into training. I was determined—and Coach Dan pushed me. But it never stopped me from living on the edge.

I first smoked weed with my siblings in middle school. Throughout high school, I'd toke up when visiting them, eyes as red as my giggly cheeks. We would wander in the woods—the trees feeling alive as their branches creaked with deep groans.

I first drank a bottle of booze with Finn—a night of music and fire. We walked back from the trail, laughing as we stumbled onto the shaky ground. We'd stare at the night sky; the stars dreamlike as the moon's glow painted the clouds silver.

I attended my first house parties in high school. Quickly getting to know strangers, we shared bottles and baggies. Someone challenged me to the gas mask bong. I concealed my face and let them light the bowl piece. The second the mask was off, I grinned—my head inflated as I collapsed from the pressure.

I was quick to get up, however.

Let me do it again.

I liked how weed and booze made me feel—out of body and childish. Despite the fact I didn't meet Coach Dan's standard, I still improved with running.

By my senior year, dozens of medals and Athlete of the Year trophies replaced the champion certificates from elementary school. I covered the letterman jacket my dad bought me with patches celebrating my achievements.

I never felt I was doing anything that harmed my running career. Even more so when my success made college seem possible.

* * *

Neither of my parents had a college degree, and it wasn't on the radar of my siblings. The idea of debt turned us away. But running gave me hope. Made the financial burden less of a worry.

I dreamt. I imagined getting a full ride into an NCAA Division I university—the top tier for athletics. I emailed coaches at Syracuse and Cornell University. One of them wrote back, telling me I needed faster race times.

Coach Dan supported the college search for my parents and me. He put together our visits. He made calls to the coaches. At some point, he encouraged a more realistic pursuit of Division III universities—the bottom tier for athletics.

Although it felt like a step back from my dream of being a professional athlete, Coach Dan kept me hopeful.

"Race times are what matters," he'd say. "You'll be a big fish in a little pond."

I understood. I'd be a lead runner at DIII versus the back of the pack at DI.

* * *

I ran faster than ever during my senior year, particularly in my final races. I had been to the New York State Track-and-Field Championships before but had yet to reach a top-three place. However, I was gaining momentum with a two-mile time of nine minutes and eleven seconds—a school and county record—and a second-place finish.

Based on states, I qualified for the five-kilometer run in the New Balance Nationals Outdoor Track-and-Field Championships. Coach Dan immediately planned the multi-day trip to Greensboro, North Carolina.

My dad traveled with us, wanting to display more awards in my room. He never missed a race. But I was in disbelief. When I looked at my competitors, I recognized that many secured scholarships to DI universities such as Princeton and Oregon.

"How did I get in this race?" I asked Coach Dan. "This is far above me."

"You're meant to be here," he replied.

That was the power of Coach Dan. He built my confidence—no doubt, no fear, and no pressure. When I stepped to the line, I wouldn't hold anything back.

I was ready to make my mark.

* * *

It was a beautiful time to run. A dark, placid sky of the spring night surrounded the track. My eyes glistened under the stadium's white bulbs. The air was warm yet cool—my energy poised.

My goal was to be in the top fifteen out of the twenty runners. Top six and All-American status, used to describe the national elite, was a dream.

The gun went off. Wearing a white singlet and black shorts, I kept a steady pace in the back. As laps passed, runners quit, staggering their steps off the track. I assumed they determined it wasn't worth it. But I was willing to hurt as much as I had to.

This race is everything.

At some point, I was in eighth place—unexpected. My patience was paying off, but I felt the pain—the hurt one feels when their stomach, throat, and muscles are about to suffocate and collapse. I still had two laps to go.

I was unsure if I had anything left in the tank. But suddenly, I felt an unexplainable force from my guts raise my breath and connect my legs. I lifted my head, preventing my body from slipping backward, and concentrated.

I had been neck and neck with another runner. When he made a move, I responded, my eyes latching onto the runners in front of me. Although they had a decent lead, I was catching them.

Ting ting ting. The final lap bell rang.

I knew I was about to be in pain unlike anything before. The closing lap was the make-it-or-break-it point, and I had to run faster than ever if I wanted sixth place.

So I did. I took off with as much speed as I could muster. I released the entirety of myself, feeling like air soaring through the creases of space and time.

The lap was a blur, white fading my vision's periphery.

Pure ecstasy.

For those sixty-three seconds, I was without worries or thoughts. I was simply there, existing in a world that moved with me. A temporary moment where I felt more alive and present than ever before. A feeling I would not forget.

In the closing hundred-meter stretch, I edged out the runner I needed to. I finished sixth place. I was an All-American.

I did belong in that race.

Raising the stakes.

* * *

I had privileges, such as in school and genetics—my discovered talent in running. I had strong social connections with Coach Dan, Finn, and Sarah. I had opportunities that helped me build skills and a work ethic—a dedicated sports community and daily structure.

I'm grateful. Without recognizing it, my circumstances supported my well-being even while I used substances and disobeyed my father. Now, I know protective factors increase the likelihood of mental health support and can reduce the impact of ACEs, and I can see how they strengthened my resilience.

As I lived with my father, Karmen married her boyfriend. Cody was in and out of jail for theft and public intoxication. Lindsay faced mental health crises that led her to the hospital and jail.

I'd hear snippets of their experiences, uncertain of how to help; I was too focused on running. Only now, after my mental illness, could I more intimately understand how disadvantages and privileges impacted our experiences.

Not everyone finds hope.

When I watch the recording of my national race, I feel joy hearing my friends and family cheering for me. But what if I wasn't successful with running? What if I didn't have Coach Dan—would I have pursued college? What if the onset of my mental illness occurred in high school?

At the time, I didn't realize how important running was to my mental health and the pressure I put on myself going into college. But now, I see it. If only I had learned how impactful life transitions can be on mental health.

What would happen if I stopped succeeding in running?

OFF-COURSE

I was young for my class. Many runners my age were a year behind me. Since my birthday was in November, my parents could've put me in school one year early or one year late.

I went to school early. If I had accomplished what I did as a senior in my junior year, I would have most likely received a DI scholarship. I would've saved money. I may have been better positioned to pursue my teenage dream of professional running.

But who knows?

Like Coach Dan, I chose SUNY Geneseo. The DIII college, thirty miles from home, was academically competitive. I increased my grade point average in the latter part of high school. But my Cs, Bs, and lower-than-average SAT scores didn't meet their standard. Thankfully, as an exceptional talent for sports, my admission was more likely.

I was accepted.

* * *

Most of my friends in college were on the team. They could loosely fit into two groups. Those in the Booze Crew chugged Natty Daddy beers regularly. Those who ran seriously abided by dry seasons, which meant no alcohol during sports.

Many were from well-off families. When visiting a friend from Westhampton on Long Island, I'd run beside shiny, luxurious homes—five times the size and forty times the cost of my dad's double-wide. I was amazed, seeing livelihoods I could only dream of or see on TV.

What would it be like to grow up here?

I didn't meet anyone with separated parents, a mixed bag of family members, and low-income status. People were shocked I had never traveled overseas and confused when I'd describe the gaps in my holiday festivities.

Only some picked up part-time jobs as I did. But I had to work if I wanted cash. I washed dishes and served sandwiches for Fusion, an on-campus restaurant. I gutted houses, mowed lawns, and squeezed in other manual labor.

Working on top of school and sports added to my separation from the team. But I still felt lucky to be there—as if I was a waiter at a high-end restaurant asked to join the customers. However, I wasn't someone who just had the chance to be there. Nor was I simply another member of the team.

I was there due to my devotion to running and my achievements. Therefore, I could not fail.

I have to win to show who I could be.

* * *

My first year proved what I was capable of. I was in the top ten freshman for cross-country nationals. I was the first freshman at my college to break the fifteen-minute barrier in the five-kilometer race. I qualified for the Junior National Track-and-Field Championships—a competition for the country's best nineteen-year-old and younger athletes.

I'm already standing out.

Campus News passed my name and picture. My parents shared the articles with my family. Likes on Facebook posts were abundant.

One teammate said, "Future national champion right here."

Everything was going as planned. Everything was perfect. Until one day.

I ran a five-mile workout on the track—each less-than-five-minute mile felt easy. But after, a stinging pain in my foot lingered for days. I sought a diagnosis and learned I had a stress fracture.

With six required weeks off, track unexpectedly ended. I missed the rest of my season. I missed my only chance at junior nationals. I was sad.

With no competition to work towards, I took advantage of my freedom from sports.

* * *

The Booze Crew organized our team's mixers with sororities and clubs. We hosted pre-games in our dorm or met with older classmates at their houses. Around midnight, we'd join dozens of drunk students meandering Geneseo's main street, grabbing a garbage plate at Pizza Paul's or stumbling into the IB—a prominent nineteen-plus dance club.

Although I was eighteen, I found my way into the club. An older teammate showed me the ropes, pulling me behind the bar and pointing to its two-story high deck. I had to use arm strength to climb, but the more challenging test was a gamble. Every other time a bouncer stood on the other side, ready to drag me out the door.

Partying was an aid—a way to forget the injury. One night, after a bottle of tequila and orange juice, I hunched over a plastic bag spewing piss-colored ooze. It was my first time blacking out, but not my last.

When I could run again, I continued my off-the-clock hobbies. I didn't feel the need to meet the *twenty-four-hour-seven-days-a-week* standard until cross-country the following fall. Plus, I wanted to embrace the college experience.

Independence. Self-exploration. No pressure.

Many nights, I'd play Cards Against Humanity or Never Have I Ever—games where others loved to express their sexual history. Eventually, a girl—short with curly brunette hair—set her dark eyes on me.

Although I was still with Sarah, a senior in high school, we saw less of each other. Our separation caused fights and a fear of what each other was doing.

"Part of me wants to be single in college," I texted a friend. "What do I do?"

Sarah saw the messages. When I approached her, she was bawling her eyes out. She then broke up with me. Just like that, a three-and-a-half-year relationship crumbled.

I regretted sending those messages. I felt guilty for being interested in another woman. But I moved on. Even though Sarah continued to talk to me—she wanted me to fight for her—I was too preoccupied with myself and what college had to offer.

* * *

The injury and my girlfriend weren't the only tests in my first year. On top of the GPA required to maintain student-athlete status, I had to consider what my studies meant.

Coach Dan recommended a communication degree to be a future coach. I heard it was easy too, so I signed on. As I took courses such as Introduction to Global Social Change, I added sociology as a second major. Something about that field connected with me. Particularly when at home in the summer, I visited Finn, and his mom inspired me to take initiative.

"These are the kids we're helping," she said, showing me a picture of a school her church built in Kenya.

She described children with physical disabilities and how beneficial physical therapy would be. I felt touched by her care for those with less privilege and saw a connection to sociology.

I need to do something.

I obtained a list of physical therapy needs from the school and formed Project Kenya to raise money. The idea of a child leaving a wheelchair due to treatment felt like something I had to do.

The right thing to do.

I worked with a student club for Project Kenya while simultaneously returning to running. We were planning a fall-themed festival. However, just as the championship races for cross-country began, I was taken out. A sharp pain twisted deep in my calf in the middle of a race, and I walked off the course limping.

Another injury. Another six weeks off.

What happened?

"Some say for highest chance of success, managing two priorities in college is ideal," Coach Dan would say. "There's sports, academics, and…"

He paused on social life.

Running was my priority. If I were to say academics took the second spot, I'd be lying—it was my social life. With my calf strain, I realized any professional effort had to be off the table.

Project Kenya faded quickly. Emails from the student club went unanswered. A local farm's donated sack of potatoes for the fall festival was left to rot. I refocused myself.

Running is the priority.

"Maybe you should limit weekly mileage to sixty," Coach Dan said. "It seems anytime you run more, an injury occurs."

I had heard higher mileage yielded better performances. Many runners would be at one hundred miles a week. But I trusted Coach Dan more than anyone. I listened when he suggested cross-training to supplement the miles I couldn't run.

I began thrashing in the college pool. My dad bought me a road bike, and I'd hit the road with sixty-mile-long rides. My training turned into a mix of swimming, running, and biking, and I prepared for my junior year of sports with a fresh mindset.

I was ready to make my mark—again.

* * *

I tried desperately to be that *twenty-four-hour-seven-days-a-week athlete.* I stayed dry. I trained more than ever. I had some success but was yet to be an All-American. Then the worst happened—again.

Another injury. Another cancellation of my sport. Another joining of the Booze Crew ranks.

Parties on top of parties. Late-night shenanigans repeated. Enough booze kept me drunk for an entire weekend. I did not understand how I kept getting injured. Even when I was going above and beyond for running, a wounded bone or muscle would cripple my spirit.

Am I destined to fail?

Something positive did happen in my junior year. I met Carrie when traveling two hours with the Booze Crew to a rival school's house party. Standing in the living room with a beer, I saw her curly blonde hair and diamond-blue eyes. At a short height, her soft smile drew me in.

"Are you on the team here?" I asked.

"Yeah," she replied. "What brings you here?"

The questions initiated our evening together. I stopped tending to the keg. She invited me to her dorm. But we didn't have sex. We talked—all night—and I felt something I hadn't had in a while: comfort.

Carrie was one of the fastest milers at her college. When I couldn't race on the weekend, I cheered my heart out from the sidelines. I'd stay over, resting my head on her shoulder. As she went to practice the next day, I anxiously waited for her return, missing her and my running shoes.

I succeeded academically more than ever when dating Carrie. My most challenging courses, such as Social Movements and Contemporary Sociological Theory, relied on paper assignments instead of exams.

In one month, I had to write sixty-plus pages, requiring many all-nighters. I went between texting Carrie and researching data to support my argument on how social change occurs. I even reduced partying, so I could focus on her and my studies.

I'm loving it.

I had never felt so dedicated to something outside of running, and it showed. I received a 3.94 GPA, the highest score I had ever received. Rather than the athletic section of campus news, the Dean's List pasted my name.

For the first time, I felt proud of my schoolwork. But I was unsure where that would get me in life. I still only saw running in my future. I never stopped thinking about my goals in the sport.

I had one cross-country season left—one more chance to succeed in a sport that meant so much to me.

What am I waiting for?

* * *

I worked hard in the summer before my last season. Every week, I trained nearly one hundred miles on the bike, three miles of swimming, and fifty miles of running. I had weight room sessions, yoga routines, core exercises, and specific workouts.

I avoided partying before the season even started. I took the *twenty-four-hour-seven-days-a-week athlete* standard to the extreme, and it showed.

With Coach Dan's encouragement, I raced triathlons—a sport combining swimming, biking, and running. After winning my first two, the USA Triathlon Collegiate Recruitment Program contacted me. An Olympian from the program that supported potential Team USA triathletes recognized I neared their qualifications.

I began to see triathlons as a potential next step for me. However, cross-country had to be first, and during the initial months, I thrived. I won several meets. I finished fifth at the NCAA DIII Pre-National Cross Country Invitational. I was running faster than ever before.

Nothing could stop me. All my hard work was coming to the surface. My team felt it. My coaches felt it. My family and Carrie felt it.

I felt it.

When nationals arrived, I was ready to make my mark.

I'm ready to be an All-American again.

Pressure intensified.

* * *

I put a lot of importance on running success. Stemming from childhood, it seemed like the only way I could prosper. Since my identity relied on the sport, my future and connection to others also did.

I wish I knew what I was going through. College had so much to offer. I'm sad I let running consume me.

Sports have unique hurdles. Defeat does not come easy. Athletic identity can be more than training and competing—it can be a lifestyle. And for me, it was. But during my athlete years, I never focused on the mental health impact of my physical injuries.

Simon Biles backing out of the 2021 Summer Olympics because of her mental health shocked the sports community. She changed the game, showing how an injury to the mind should be considered a reason to step back.

I wish I had known that athletes could take this path. When injuries disrupted my athletic career, I avoided my feelings by partying. I never examined my struggle to be that *twenty-four-hour seven-days-a-week athlete*. Instead, I developed a vicious cycle of hard work, failure, and self-medication, adding more pressure on each season to compensate for the lost time.

I now see how desperate I felt to hold onto my identity. I didn't know how to assess my wellness or need for support. I didn't know discussing my mental health could reduce stress since no one I knew talked about it.

Anyone can face mental health challenges and become unwell without knowing. If I had recognized how we all have mental health and approached my challenges differently, like I do now, maybe I would've gotten help earlier.

What if my academics or Project Kenya became more of a focus throughout college? What if I didn't get injured or learned how to respond to failure with healthier coping—would I have partied less? What if it was common practice to get mental health support when injured?

With cross-country nationals around the corner, the stress was extreme. I now realize how my future did not have to rely on a single race—I never needed sports to live well. But at that time, running was everything.

If I did not accomplish what I wanted, what would come next?

THE FINISH LINE

The day in Mason, Ohio was cold. Patches of the ground were wet from snow. The sky was cloudy, and the air was bitter. Cross-country nationals were always on the brink of fall and winter, but the team prepared like any other race.

I started in a good position. The gun shot, and I leaped to the front, joining dozens of sticky bodies. Although the muddied ground caused my spiky shoes to slosh and stagger, I was focused.

The first two miles went by fast. I remained near the front. But when the halfway mark hit—a defining moment for a runner's strength—something changed.

The ground began plastering my toes. My body dropped back. I felt unsteady.

I looked ahead to see grassy hills and curves saturated with deep footprints. A major competitor of mine then zoomed past me as if I was walking. My sight fell in reverse.

"You got this! You can stay with him," a teammate chanted from the sidelines.

No—no, I did not. My legs were running out of gas. For the remainder of the race, I lost my grip.

Runner after runner passed me. My feet dragged in muck and gunk. My determination suffocated in the cold, wet air.

When the finish line neared, my dad, Coach Dan, and teammates stood by, cheering. But instead of inspiration, I felt defeated.

I stumbled into a one hundred and first place. Close to where I finished my first year—far from what I had achieved in my last high school race.

No one on my team did well. We all crashed and burned. I was able to celebrate something though. The day before nationals, I turned twenty-one.

I can drink legally.

* * *

I bought my teammates and me booze for the bus ride home. I texted my friends, whom I partied with, amping up the evening for some serious drinking. Since I didn't want to remember nationals, I would surely make it a night to remember.

Just like the race, I started strong. Beer after beer in my hands—a satisfying crack preempted the flow of crisp suds down my gullet. With the volume of booze, my legs wobbled. But I was determined to drink more.

The night was going by fast. From pregame to party…to maybe another party…I found myself in Kelly's—a dive bar I could finally go to.

It was loud. Sticky bodies rubbed against each other. Faces blurred. Like the second half of the race, my body dissipated in a sloppy stream.

"To Cohen. Happy twenty-first birthday!" A friend toasted.

I guzzled a shot, liquor burning my innards. Almost immediately, my sight fell in reverse. The sweat of human flesh faded.

Lights reflecting off the wooden bar turned black. Incoherent chatter went silent.

My world ended, and the morning unknowingly came. I failed at making it a night to remember. Deep down, I wanted to forget.

* * *

My failure with running reached its peak after my final cross-country race. What made me ambitious and dedicated—a son, teammate, and friend to be proud of—now did the opposite.

How can I come back from this?

I drank more than I prepared for the following track season. Once I began to train, I felt a pin-pointed pain in my shin.

Another injury. Why?

As usual, my coaches suggested time off, and I listened. But what I didn't do was assess the pain any further—the pain in my leg nor the pain inside. I didn't even pursue cross-training to remain fit. Instead, I left the sport and indulged in the college experience.

I chugged beers. I smoked bowls dense with weed. Consuming it all at once, I let myself feel the complete freedom of a student who just wanted to have fun and party.

I'm good at it.

I could slug a three-beer boot in less than ten seconds. I could rip several strikeouts—a shot of liquor, a hit off a bong, and a beer chug while holding my breath the entire time. I could flip my legs above a keg and slurp Genny Light out its spigot until fizz shot out of my nose.

"Twenty-seven! Twenty-eight! Twenty-nine!" my friends chanted as if I was about to get a personal record in a race.

I'm still someone special.

* * *

Going to bars and parties turned into a weekday thing. Opportunities to meet new people and other girls happened almost every night.

I had been with Carrie for a year, getting her romantic gifts and saying those three words daily. But our love broke as swiftly as I quit running.

I was at fault. One night at a house party, I was talking to a girl with brown eyes and straight black hair. The next thing I knew, she pushed my back against a wall and pressed her lips onto mine. I took on the pleasure for five minutes too long.

The stranger wanted to go further, but I stopped. I didn't want to cheat. I felt guilty for what I had done and called Carrie right after.

"I'm sorry, babe. I didn't mean to."

"Why didn't you stop sooner," she sobbed. "I can't be with you anymore."

I felt horrible and quickly regretted calling her. Maybe I could have communicated my feelings better. Maybe we could've worked it out. But instead, I lost her just like that and turned to what I came to love—non-stop partying.

Like Sarah, Carrie continued talking to me, wanting me to fight for her. We even hooked up a couple of times. But I was changing and being selfish—*again*.

* * *

My failure with running fractured other parts of my life. On top of my athletic career and relationships crumbling, I received the lowest GPA ever.

But it's okay.

All I needed to feel fine was weed, beer, and friends to join me. Even when my lack of care brought toxic moments.

Many nights, I messaged a friend's ex-girlfriend in an attempt to hook up with her. I broke a bro code with no disgrace. I was single, she was single, and I was losing sight of my moral reasoning.

On another occasion, I stole Oakley sunglasses at a party. My irritation with the shallowness of over-priced eyewear revealed itself—as if the resentment for those with more privilege came to the forefront of my mind.

I wanted to break all the rules—fight the man. However, I was beginning to not feel remorse for treating others horribly. I wasn't even capable of treating myself well.

Who the hell am I?

* * *

Coach Dan, who had been hired as an assistant coach for SUNY Geneseo, and I rarely spoke after I stopped attending practice. I most likely dismissed him if he reached out. Since I was not training, we didn't need to talk. But in the summer before my final year of college—I had planned to take a fifth year—he had the biggest race of his life. I chose to go.

Coach Dan spent years training for the 2015 Lake Placid Ironman Regional Championships. His goal was to qualify for the Ironman World Championships. But it wasn't just for him. He was dedicating the race to his sister who had recently passed away.

When I arrived at the course, the atmosphere was magical. Dozens of people were there to support him. Messages such as "Do it for Molly" and "Believe and Achieve" were written on shirts, signs, and cement roads. Chants of his name echoed throughout the Adirondack Mountains.

I felt inspired—something I hadn't had since cross-country ended. I ran around the course, finding spots where I'd catch a glimpse of my hero.

"Come on, Coach, you got this!" My cheers sounded familiar.

He noticed me when transitioning onto the bike portion of the race. Our eyes met—determination sparkled on his face. He then raised a finger and pointed at me.

I didn't need words to understand what he meant. I felt it.

Coach Dan wants me back.

As the race finished, and he achieved his goal, I wanted to be back too.

* * *

I moved forward with my fifth-year plan. I was to be a volunteer assistant coach in cross-country and train for track in the spring. However, I was a liar.

I ran some miles here and there. I joined a couple of workouts. But something felt off. I wasn't enjoying it anymore.

I smoked weed daily, spending eighty bucks a week to meet my demands. Any savings from years of work at Fusion disappeared just like that.

I smoked while driving. I smoked before and after work and class. I smoked when helping to coach practice once a week. At a precise moment, while the team ran mile repeats in a large field, I'd pull out my bowl and sneak hits.

No one knows.

For races, something a coach should undoubtedly be at, I tried finding excuses not to go. I may have gone to one or two of them. When everyone rallied for the championship portion of the season, I appeared late, stoned, and hungover, standing by the sidelines, trying to hide.

No one sees me.

False promises of being there for track kept Coach Dan at bay. But others attempted to make a point to me.

"Stop smoking that fucking weed," a different coach had said.

"When will you be back?" a teammate asked.

Nothing but statements associated with running. However, I wasn't coming back. I was one hundred feet behind my prior self.

I was nothing but a *twenty-four-hour-seven-days-a-week pothead.*

* * *

Outside of cross-country, my responsibilities remained the same. Go to class. Show up to work. Be home whenever.

I had moved back to my dad's because the friends I had lived with left. They moved on with their lives, going to professional jobs or graduate school. I slowly regretted my decision to stay a fifth year. So, I smoked more.

I had to be sly with weed at my dad's. As far as he knew, I was doing everything right. But if he caught me with pot, it'd be a game changer.

My car—an old Subaru Outback—became my favorite place to be. I would drive into the woods to smoke on my own. I'd visit my friends and family who smoked with me.

The more I smoked, the better I felt. Nothing was wrong.

The world is fascinating.

I paid close attention to how people socialize. Their movements and dialogue. Their emotions and thoughts. I did the same when I viewed TV and social media.

I saw the Disney film *Inside Out* with my sister Casie. Leaning back in a comfy reclining chair, the colors and sounds of the big screen entranced me. The characters inside the little girl's head, who represented emotions and used a control panel to manage her feelings, created questions for me.

How are our emotions created? What do they do for us? Are there forces inside my head controlling me?

Perhaps a trippy thought. One people might associate with the effects of weed or drugs such as shrooms or LSD. However, even as I left the theater and the high subsided, I couldn't get the ideas from the movie out of my head.

Do I have control over myself? Or is everything determined by something else?

For the first time, I had to decipher whether life was a movie. Things were starting to feel different.

* * *

I had been desperate for a future goal since running was no longer in the picture. As the new year approached, I explored the unique thoughts flowing in my mind.

One day, I had an exhilarating idea.

How about writing a movie?

I had been piecing together what I believed was a powerful story. In the narrative, the audience would follow the main character, a collegiate distance runner. The young athlete made so much progress because of how good the coach was—their relationship being the focus of the setup. But as adverse situations kept happening to him, he unexpectedly stopped training.

The plot could include failure, relationship issues, and substance misuse. It could involve social problems such as poverty or the pressures of partying in college. Eventually, the athlete and coach's relationship would be torn apart.

Until one day.

The coach had spent years training for a world-class race of daring difficulty. When he achieved his goal, his inspiration would fuel the athlete's return. The movie would end with them running beside each other once again, training together for years to come—happier ever after.

IronDan would be the title. An instant hit—I felt it.

My future is certain.

* * *

I gained a strong sense of motivation and purpose again. I spent hours in the library studying screenplay literature and writing the story. A couple of times, I skipped work because I—*my brain*—had sudden ideas I didn't want to forget.

Screenplay writing was my newfound dream. A lofty career I desired after graduation and a fantasy that allowed me to imagine a life I stopped pursuing. However, when I took my final courses to graduate, things changed again.

I began Humanities in the spring when my world turned upside down. Fueled by the class content, I started to ask heavier questions than what *Inside Out* sparked for me. Ideas that grew bigger than the screenplay. Much bigger.

What entered with this diversion were challenges unlike I ever experienced before.

Who am I?

Running adrift.

* * *

The failure I felt in my last cross-country race broke me completely. I was devastated and lost. My partying increased and toxic traits emerged. As my health and well-being deteriorated, early signs and symptoms of mental illness filtered through the cracks.

One in five people are predisposed to mental illness, and I'm one of them. Maybe, if more people knew that, we'd focus more on addressing it. Maybe my illness would have been noticed, and I would've gotten help earlier. Maybe I would not be feeling frustrated with how uncommon mental health education is.

So, what are some basics?

Signs and symptoms differ. Signs are what people recognize in someone's behavior, thoughts, or feelings, such as a noticeable change in relationships and responsibilities. Symptoms are perceived by the person affected and vary per diagnosis, such as mania in bipolar or psychosis in schizophrenia.

Signs don't always mean someone has mental illness; they may just be unwell. But that shouldn't stop anyone from getting help.

My willingness to leave a sport I cherished and the drastic relationship changes with Coach Dan and Carrie were signs. However, since I maintained responsibilities with school and work, I may have come off as okay—the signs were harder to see.

Since I did not understand mental health, I wouldn't notice the symptoms. Now, I know my bizarre thoughts after *Inside Out* resembled early psychosis—a disconnection from reality. My movie writing obsession resembled early mania—a euphoric mood with grandiose thoughts.

My marijuana and alcohol misuse were unusual, and others noticed. But I used it to cope—to self-medicate and continue avoiding painful feelings. I now see how substances exacerbated my mental health challenges, but I also know they alone didn't incite the illness.

What if a friend or Coach Dan pursued an open conversation about why I stopped attending practice? What if I reached out to someone about what I was going through? What if I or those close to me better understood mental health—would I have been more likely to seek support through treatment instead of self-medicating?

But no one stepped in and urged me to get help. Sadly, I wasn't equipped for what was ahead.

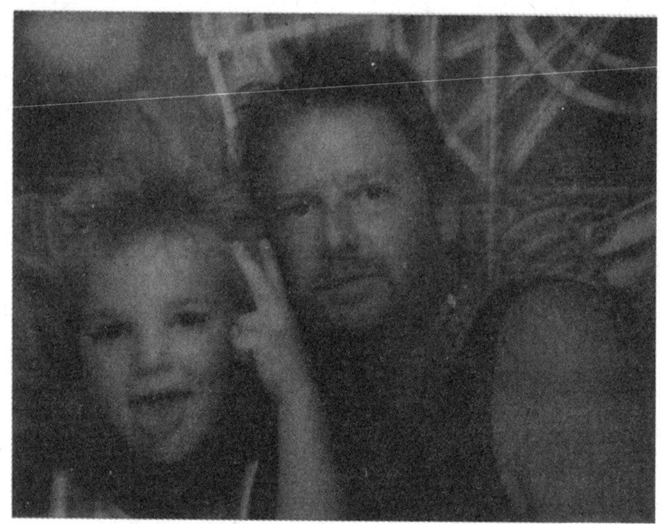

Cohen and Dad

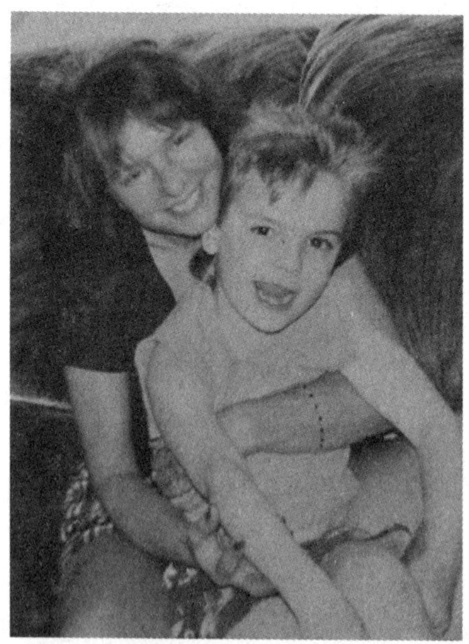

Cohen and Mom

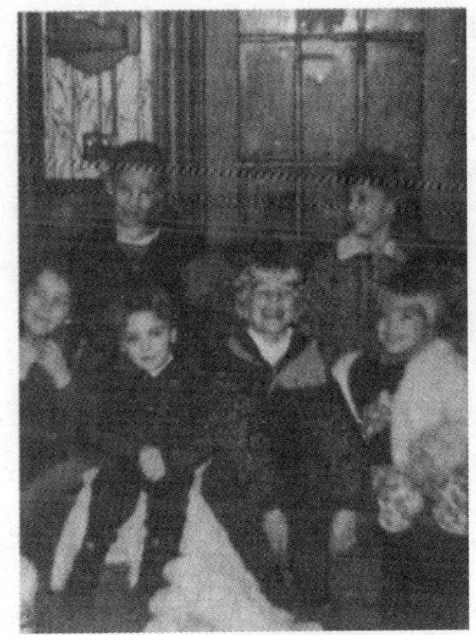

Cohen and his siblings

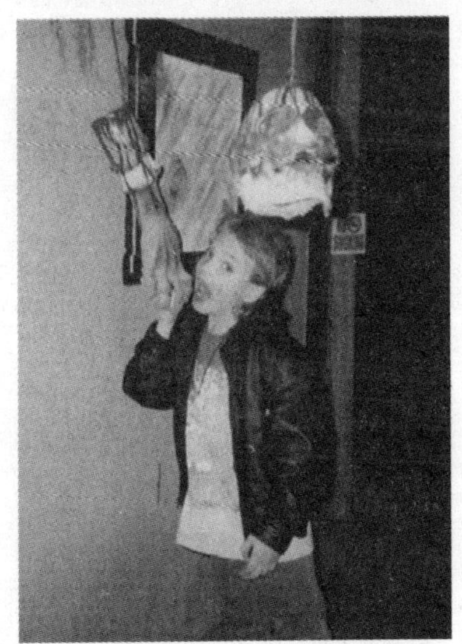

Cohen at a haunted house

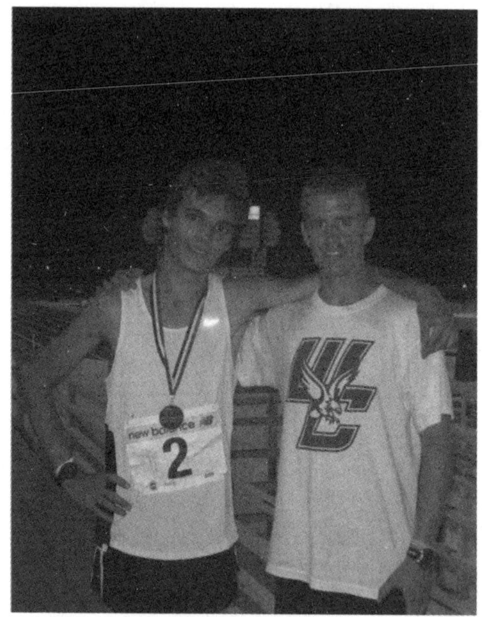

Coach Dan and Cohen at New Balance Nationals

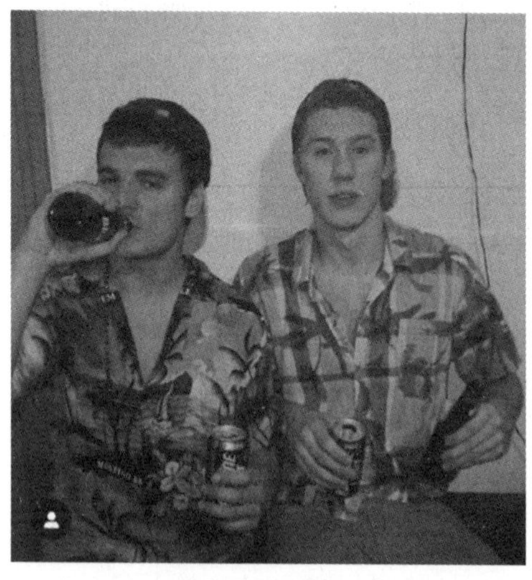

Cohen at a party

PART II

THE UNKNOWN

The professor of Humanities stood tall when he spoke. He was an aged man with white hair, a long beard, and square eyeglasses. His classroom of gray walls and arranged chairs felt sterile and orderly. But his voice caused a commotion in my mind.

I had been high in many classes but never felt like I did in Humanities. Something was different.

In one class, the professor towered over a student, staring at their Starbucks coffee with wide eyes. I followed suit, noticing the soft brown liquid sway in its clear rounded cup. Although a simple device, the cup had such precise carrying capabilities.

The professor made assumptions about the coffee and how it existed in his fingers. He mentioned a person far away harvesting a plant, a factory creating the cup, the company's advertisements seen by us, and so on.

He then questioned.

"Why do you drink this?" he asked. "How certain are you of how it came to be here?"

The simple inquiry into the nature of the coffee provoked my pondering thoughts.

I want to know more.

* * *

In another class, the professor played an instrument called the Hurdy Gurdy. Its rustic wood, molded into a roundish square shape, looked like it was from an ancient ruin, resembling an early version of a guitar. The rod turned at its base created a unique and archaic sound.

I didn't know what to expect when the Professor directed us to pay close attention to his finger movements and observe the sound waves radiating off the strings.

"Let go of all thoughts," he said. "Focus exclusively on the here and now and the rhythmic nature of these sounds."

The strum of a medieval-like tune captivated the classroom with graceful harmonies. A floating sensation lifted the air. The glow of lights encircled me.

I felt a serene balance and ambiance—a sense of mind-and-body connectedness and, yet, a separation of thought into what I was doing and why. For a brief moment, I thought I could transport myself to the Middle Ages.

I wanted to stay here. I wanted the moment to go on forever. But when the professor's fingers reeled back, I snapped into my familiar state. I became what I didn't want to be again.

"How did that make you feel?" the Professor asked.

I kept my answer quiet. But I felt a sense of understanding—as if the answers to my uncertainty with life were somehow interwoven in the playing of the instrument.

Something made sense.

But what is it?

* * *

My thoughts picked up the pace with every class. I began crafting ideas about the topics discussed, letting the professor's voice stimulate my thoughts. Instead of looking forward, I'd be hunched over my desk, writing feverishly in my notebook. Eventually, I was the one asking questions.

"How can humans, who have been smart enough to travel to the moon, not be able to achieve world peace?" I asked.

The room fell silent. I sensed the students' speechlessness after hearing my voice. Although the professor didn't have much of an answer, his facial expression told me he was impressed.

I seemed to be onto something.

Something important.

In another class, we had to review an interpretation of social justice with a partner. The girl who sat in front of me, turned around, eager to interact. But before she could say anything, I spoke.

"Isn't it about the greater good? Does an individual's opinion really matter?"

I rambled on, believing I had made arguments that proved my point. She didn't respond—or, at least, I didn't hear her. I just saw tears in her eyes.

She gets it.

* * *

Over time, the classroom wasn't big enough for my evolving worldviews. I began analyzing every element of all things and practiced being present outside of class.

I'd hike in the woods, sit on a rock, and examine white water drops from a cliff into a still, dark pool. Everything—the slanted stone, the trees nearby, the open space for the water to fall—had a physical calculation one could figure out. A natural phenomenon of shapes and shadows turned into numbers and patterns.

At night, I would lie under the covers, pretend I was in the center of space, and watch *Friends* on my smartphone for hours. I'd forget my life—my story—and live in those of Joey, Chandler, and the rest. When Ross and Rachel kissed for the first time, it felt like her lips were on mine. A natural phenomenon of social interaction turned into entertainment.

What is it about the human connection we can't figure out?

When I was with people—actual people—I had difficulty being present with them. I couldn't be bothered by their unnecessary stress with the weather or what someone said on social media. I distanced myself from these distractions and encouraged others to do the same.

"Can we ignore our phones for the next thirty minutes?" I'd say. "Tell me, what can we do at this moment to forget the stress?"

Sometimes they engaged with me in the present. But removing all distractions wasn't easy. A few minutes would pass, and they'd be staring at their smartphone again. Or they'd talk about something complex and irrelevant to our presence, which then created tension.

I dismissed their stress by recognizing it and shifting my thoughts to be in tune with the present. The more I practiced, the easier it was. Soon enough, I could be present all of the time.

I wanted everyone to feel the same. But I didn't have the words to express what I was going through. It felt like I could grasp the thoughts while, at the same time, I couldn't.

* * *

One afternoon, a few months into the spring semester, I traveled to Books & Bites, a popular café in the campus library. Intending to observe the area, I ordered coffee, sat, and settled my mind and body.

The room had green and brown tones. Its tall windows produced a beam of fresh sunlight. Chattering voices and dish clangor rippled across the space.

Some faces were glued to black smartphones—their eyes and hands stuck to the tiny devices. Others looked towards one another, exchanging contact with the food they ate. Few felt silent, even though they were always doing something such as reading a book or cleaning a tabletop.

Each moment had some form of movement. Someone's limb in motion. Light-shifting color. A speck of dust floating.

Everything felt never-ending.

All these things exist in the same space as one and, yet, multiple different things.

The more I observed, the more I felt a simultaneous connection and disconnection.

Everything is so fascinating…

The infinite faces. The chaotic melody of sounds. My presence.

But…

No one knew me. No one knew me although I was right in front of them. If I wanted to speak to another, I'd have had to break down a perceived wall.

Why?

No one in the cafe focused on their presence. Not a single person stopped what they were doing with their hands or mouth to be still and connect with what surrounded them.

They just kept going and going, absorbed by the reality made up in their head.

But I'm breaking the mold.

I saw things hidden within the present. I shaped the silence. I moved the world; it didn't move me.

Within this stillness—this transparency between existence and life—I needed answers.

What does it mean to be here?

* * *

I sat in the cafe for another hour, interpreting. I identified that I could experience and perceive. I could be with what was in my immediate presence, think about what was not, and have a sensation with both.

I sniffed my coffee—tiny molecules in the air touching my nose. I pressed its liquid to my tongue—a bitter, creamy taste. I let it flow down my throat—my innards coated in warmth.

I thought about my first time drinking coffee in the library as a freshman. Not only did it help energize me to finish a late-night paper, but I remembered enjoying its flavor and aroma—just as much as I did now.

Would my experience with coffee be the same if it weren't for my perceived memory? Do things outside our presence impact the present?

I understood my belief that the building I sat in was built by humans I never met. I understood that I believed others in the café were students like me, living a similar life. I understood where my home and car were located. But I couldn't actually see them.

Are they figures painted in my head?

Was it possible my car and home would be gone after I left the café?

Would I walk into pure darkness if I stepped outside the doors—as if being here meant I was nowhere else?

I knew what to expect when drinking coffee—my memory ensured that. But was it possible my existence had just begun, and that memory was erected in my mind?

Are memories beliefs too?

I felt a bit of truth soak through the skin tightened around my body. Ideas of oddity and absurdity washed over me as I watched myself from above.

Like the film shot that zooms out from a character, my mind was the camera, and my body shrunk in the frame. Soon enough, I was a tiny Cohen—existing at a singular point in space, drinking coffee in Books & Bites.

Frozen in time.

On the precipice of delusion.

* * *

A few days after the café, I had a breakthrough. When analyzing my Humanities notes, all things suddenly made sense.

The world is this way because of that…we humans are like that because of this…the reason for everything is there….

I felt exhilarated.

But how to communicate this?

It didn't take me long to figure it out.

A theory to explain all things.

A universal, objective truth no one could deny. One that would elevate our beings and resolve every issue in society.

I opened my notebook to a clean sheet of white paper. I wrote the question about world peace. I wrote questions about existence and life. I described my view of human connection—what it meant to be present and have thoughts.

On and on, I deciphered. On and on, I drew lines and added symbols to connect ideas—editorial marks that scattered beyond the margins. By the end, the single page looked like a puzzle.

I got it.

The more I dug into my ideas, the more I felt they had existed in me for my entire life—locked beneath the deep-seated matter of my brain's neurons. I simply needed to unearth the hidden chest and guide its essence out.

I was born to discover this theory.

My childhood. My rising stardom as an athlete. My ability to find new outlets of appreciation.

I was someone different.

Someone special.

* * *

My vision of cracking the code and saving humanity became inescapable. Empowered by the idea of sprinting across the finish line, I had to achieve my goal—on top this time.

But what's next?

It didn't take long to figure it out.

Share.

The need for others to understand my theory felt as important as figuring it out. So, when driving home from a Saint Patrick's Day party, I discussed it with a friend for the first time.

The night was long, and the morning was gray. He was hungover. I was hungover. But that didn't stop me from talking for two hours straight.

I described my story with IronDan. I told him about Humanities—the professor and his insightfulness. My tone then shifted.

"How do we know what is true?" I asked. "What do you think is true?"

"I…uh…" he uttered.

"There has to be a way to figure it out," I added. "The reason starts from the beginning…the root of all things."

On and on, I rambled. On and on—my train of thought was fast and unrelenting as I bounced from one idea to the next.

He couldn't get a word in. I controlled the space. Eventually, he stopped listening.

I wanted validation. I wanted to be heard. But I didn't get it.

By the time the car ride ended, however, I thought of someone who might.

The professor of Humanities.

* * *

Humanities helped me see how I never questioned anything. I never asked how I came to be, or what was the certainty of anything I had ever been told.

Who was I, what was I doing, where was I going, and why?

But now, I was figuring it out. I was going to figure it out. I just needed someone to listen.

What was supposed to be my final semester of undergraduate college became a springtime of awakening—of thinking differently. As quickly as the snow changed to rain and the grass turned green, my fundamental understanding of reality became unknown.

I had to know.

A sickly fixation.

* * *

My mental health declined throughout college. It had been a year since my last cross-country race. Since no one, including myself, addressed my early signs and symptoms, they worsened.

If someone intervened at this time or before, I don't think I would have embraced treatment like I do now. People wait an average of eleven years to receive help since the onset of mental illness.

Why?

What would it be like if we ignored physical illness for that long? Imagine someone coughing blood. We know that can be a sign of a greater physical health challenge. So, we talk about it.

We ask questions. How long it has been happening? Do you have any other symptoms? And so on.

We may speculate. Chest infection. Lung cancer. But we don't make any diagnosis because we're not doctors. Instead, we suggest professional help even if they've already thought of it.

Could we do something similar with mental health?

If I were to go back in time, I'd tell myself to seek professional help. It's not healthy to obsess over a theory, spend a lot of time alone, or envision cracking the code to save humanity.

I'd urge my friend, who I talked with for two hours straight, to tell my father, "Hey, I think Cohen might be unwell. He isn't acting like himself." Maybe he was concerned but didn't know how to help.

I'd tell my father to pay attention to my behavior and question what I was up to. Maybe if he asked me about schoolwork, he would have learned about my bizarre thoughts with the theory.

If any of this happened, maybe, just maybe, I would've gotten help sooner and treatment would've had a higher chance of success. Because I didn't know the path my mental illness would take. Without intervention, it would run its course.

But what would that be?

MANIC INSIGHT

It was a late Tuesday afternoon. I sat in the same bustling café of the school library. In front of me, my notebook displayed the single page with scattered notes.

The professor was arriving soon. For the first time, I'd share my work with a person I considered an expert in philosophy. Knowing what it would mean if he approved, I felt inspiration—an optimistic desire for grand achievement.

I observed while waiting. Shades of light spread throughout the café, displaying the never-ending details of a forever-moving place. Chattering students focused on trivial things, missing the beauty of what I was seeing.

A high-definition TV in the upper corner kept grabbing my attention. I could slightly hear the projection of mismatched sounds. Its spirited hues of blue, red, black, and white matched what I saw around me.

I felt the vividness of my presence—a lively force I was ready to emit with intense thrill. It was like the blood of my heart boiled, and my rib cage was set to erupt. But I kept my cool.

Even though every movement and sound of the café was stimulating, I felt at peace. An ideal space to witness and discuss the chaotic yet simple order of life and existence.

Perfection.

* * *

"I see the world differently," I told the professor the second he joined me.

His eyes, soft and wet, indicated some form of understanding. But before he could respond, I took off with my ideas—my voice racing with my mind.

"This is that, and that is this, and this is that, and that is this..." I rambled, believing my words to be efficient and understood.

Eventually, the professor snapped his fingers in front of my face. I immediately shut up.

"What is the purpose of our meeting?" he asked.

I was thrown off, thinking I had made it clear. I told him I wanted guidance with my theory—a theory to explain everything—a theory that would bring every person together.

"You would achieve what great thinkers have tried to discover for thousands of years," I recall him saying. "It may be impossible. Some say there is a combination of words out there that can change the entirety of the world, but no one really knows."

I sensed a persisting uncertainty in his response.

But I have to know. I want to succeed in the challenge.

In a change of topic, the professor pointed at my coffee cup.

"How did that come to be?" he asked.

I turned to the TV in the corner and mentioned how the news had no relevance to our immediate presence. I reinforced how I could not comprehend what the anchors were saying, yet I saw this image of them.

Speaking more steadily than before, I discussed other ideas from my notebook. The professor's attentiveness made me feel like he was starting to approve. At some point, he mentioned the need for concise statements.

"Like $e = mc^2$," he said. "That changed science forever."

I understand.

I had to summarize my theory into a precise and powerful statement. A sentence as condensed as Einstein's Theory of Relativity equation.

* * *

I left the café feeling as though I was given a mission. My mind and body felt as fresh as the spring air. Confidence coursed through my veins with each step.

When I neared my car, ready to leave campus, a hand touched my shoulder. I turned to see the professor—eyes wider than ever.

"How is it possible for you to know all of this?" he asked.

Simple.

With a fierce poke to my forehead, I told him my thoughts were reaching peak performance—how I trained my mind throughout my entire life for this.

Without a response, the professor disappeared like a momentary vision. His last-minute presence—a moment burned in my memory—validated my thoughts of being someone special.

I have my destiny.

* * *

I wanted to summarize my theory into one sentence by the next Humanities class. With it being on Thursday, I had two days to achieve my goal.

The evening after meeting with the professor looked typical. My dad sat in his recliner—laid back, feet perched, eyes glazing over the TV's changing pictures. I was in my usual spot on the couch.

Although my body presented its ordinary self, my mind was elsewhere.

World-changing words...world-changing words...

In what world could one create world-changing words?

As I contemplated the sentence, the space before me dissolved into clay. Once smooth and soft, details glittered like gold in a gold mine.

Colors shimmered—dull stars united with sharp diamonds. The big screen—a seventy-inch 4K TV—sparkled like a magic portal into another dimension. Its audio, amplified by suppressed airwaves from which a surround sound system roared, vibrated in sync with my heartbeat. Each minute felt thirty seconds longer.

Like musical notes bound to the bars of rhythm, I believed I was meant to feel this way.

But how to write the perfect harmony?

I struggled. I knew it wouldn't be easy, but the battle brewing within began to feel impossible.

Is this an endless task? Is the professor trying to determine if I could succeed in the ultimate test? Or is he making me realize there is no answer—no way to do it—and, perhaps, that's the answer?

My mind moved as fast as my legs used to run. Even though it felt like I was being pushed to the boundary of what was possible and not, I knew one thing.

I wouldn't give up. I wouldn't succumb to the pressure. I wouldn't fail again.

I imagined myself in the ideal race, recalling what it was like to be patient and smart. I'd start in a position where others guided me. I'd use the course to my advantage and run the tangents—straight lines getting me to point B the fastest.

When the finish neared, the difficulty would blind me. But no matter how worn out and withered I was, I would not stop.

Within this train of thought, my body's magnetism bound me to the earth, and I learned my next step. I had to summarize my theory in a paragraph first.

Perhaps then, the sentence would be easier.

* * *

I gained momentum as the evening turned into the night. Thinking in my most grandiose state, I focused on concise yet big-picture language—vast words to explain vast things. Soon enough, I had the first sentence.

Throughout all of time and human existence, we humans live on a bodily consumed Earth.

That was it. I felt it. A flood of understanding brimmed the edges of my mind, and the rest of the paragraph flowed as a river does to polish its rocks.

I jumped off the couch. I slammed my notebook on the table in our living room. I began saying everything out loud, pacing around as I pieced critical words together with my fingers.

"We consume. We have perspective!" I said. "How we choose to see ourselves and each other…"

"What are you working on?" my dad asked, forcing me to pause.

"Um…something for Humanities," I said. "I gotta have it done by Thursday."

He quickly ignored me, keeping his attention on the TV. Anything for college was obviously important.

I reread my paragraph's first draft, making changes. Over and over, I read and edited, tightening my words while tossing incorrect papers on the floor. I had to ensure no mistakes.

"To understand the true nature of things, shouldn't I be in the true nature of earth as my natural self? Or else how would I know?" I said. "Shouldn't I be naked in the middle of the woods?"

My dad looked half-puzzled and half-annoyed that I stood in front of the TV. But I continued. I continued stepping further into the relationship between myself and the environment around me.

"Look, I'm connected to the floor from my head to my feet," I added. "The floor I stand on is connected to that table. All the way up the table is that red cup. Why can't I move that cup with my mind? We're connected."

For a brief moment, with heavy intensity, I pierced my eyes into the cup and tried to move it. It didn't move. I tried again but failed.

With my fast movement and hasty voice, my dad wasn't keeping up.

"Cohen, can you move?" he asked. "You're blocking the TV."

I listened.

The answers are on the tip of my tongue.

Not a moment later, I figured it out.

* * *

After cleaning up the drafts of my paragraph, I took out a clean, crisp white sheet. Paying attention to every line I drew, I wrote the final version in my best handwriting and underlined words of particular importance—things that needed further explanation.

> *Throughout all of time and human existence, we humans live on a bodily-consumed Earth. An Earth that is morphing from the different perspectives of each and every human. With each and every human comes a morphing mind. If we, in mind-and-body, spend our limited time with every-one-and-everything, we can teach ourselves and each other to want love in all that exists through God. Therefore, once we as individuals have morphed our-body-and-mind to want this love, we find peace among our society. With peace comes a heavenly Earth.*

I delicately placed the paper in my blue folder labeled French. I never used it for class, and the color blue felt safe in securing this imperative work.

Whew.

I let my mind rest. The world's weight lifted off me. Thinking I accomplished what I needed for the night, I felt a sweeping tiredness.

"Goodnight, Dad," I said, heading to bed.

A minute later, he knocked on my door. Before I could respond, he opened it and stepped in.

"Are you okay, Cohen?" he asked.

"Yes, of course I am."

How am I not okay?

I was one step closer to the sentence that would change it all. The sentence that would be the foundation of humanity-saving glory.

The sentence of my destiny.
Foreseeable fallout.

* * *

The following morning arrived as fast as my thoughts raced through the night. I waited until my dad left to have the house to myself.

Once the front door shut—the indicator I was alone—I rushed out of my bedroom. Before anything else, I opened the blue folder.

One sentence. One sentence.

I didn't forget about my job at Fusion during lunchtime. But I had no lack of confidence. I could think about the sentence while performing my duty as a sandwich maker.

I rolled meat. I stocked veggies. I cut fluffy loaves of bread, pondering what words might go into the sentence.

Presence...mind...body....

My palm on the brown crust was soft. My fingers firmly held the steel knife. Thoughts kept coming. At the same time, my effortlessly-guided being felt present with all things.

People lined up and ordered. I flattened the bread, laying yellow cheese side by side on the meat of darker colors. I grabbed a peel and shimmied the entity to the next step.

I opened an oven of rectangular shapes with ease. No need to count—I hit a button and watched a thirty-second countdown.

Symmetrical precision.

New smells aromatized the air. I lined the melted cheese with two tomatoes, a handful of lettuce, and five straight streams of garlic aioli. A simple fold assembled the final substance. Then it all disappeared—taken in the hands of another being who walked out of my view.

As I formed many sandwiches, I recognized how my hands and feet moved with accuracy. My thoughts, actions, and feelings connected with one another, those of the customer, and all things that allowed the moments to be made.

The mechanisms of my world were in sync.

Amazing.

* * *

The lunch shift passed in the blink of an eye. When dinner time arrived, I had yet to discover the sentence. However, I had an idea that would be my saving grace.

Throughout childhood, I looked up to Finn and his intellectual ability. I admired his thoughts about what was important in life. Thinking he could help, I reached out. We planned to meet that evening.

Driving home from campus, I pictured Finn and I conversing in-depth about the meaning of life, trying to locate the truth through our interlacing minds. It made sense someone I had a personal connection with would advise me on the sentence.

We started the evening with a small campfire in his backyard. As usual, we sipped on beers. I tapped on my *cajón*—a box designed for gentle drumming—and he strummed his guitar. Our wooden instruments radiated warmth as the fire's orange glow contrasted with the moonlight.

I fell into a deep comfort while playing. My mind was as silent as my mouth had been all day. But the moment our hands and beat-tapping feet stopped, I could no longer hold back. My mountain of thoughts erupted like a volcano.

I left my blue folder at home. So, instead of discussing the paragraph, I addressed music.

"What makes people love music?" I asked Finn.

Before he could respond, I answered.

"It must be the elements and physics of sound vibrations and their patterns. Its perfect balance creates that pleasing feeling with people," I said. "Music is essentially science."

I sensed Finn's sudden perplexity—a similar look to my dad's face the night before.

"I've put my heart into music," he said, irritated. "It's art."

Standing from his stool—tall with broad shoulders, double my size—he instructed me into his house. He wanted to watch *Into the Wild*—a movie I hadn't seen—because I reminded him of the main character.

The movie follows Chris McCandless, a college-aged man, who left his traditional lifestyle and career to embark on a journey into the wilderness. He removes himself from unnecessary possessions, burns money, and goes to Alaska alone.

As the movie began, I immediately noticed similarities between Chris and me. He was an American man with brown curly hair. He was a cross-country runner. Our ideas of the world seemed to be the same.

"I don't need a new car. I don't want a new car," he said to his parents, talking about his old, but in good shape, Datsun. "I don't want anything—these things, things, things."

Eventually, the movie felt directed to me—as if I was meant to see it at that time and location. When Chris started hiking in the woods, I couldn't help but comment.

"If he truly wanted to be in the wild, wouldn't he have to get rid of his watch…and even his clothes?" I said to Finn.

"Why don't you just sit down and watch the movie?" he replied with exasperation.

Apparently, I'd been pacing around the room and talking non-stop since the start of it. I didn't remain seated for long though.

In one scene, Chris argued with a border patrol attendant about not having a passport. His face spiraled with confusion—like he genuinely didn't understand how a human couldn't walk on land.

…

He's right, though. Right?

Absurdity punched me in my gut. In those seconds, it felt like I became as delusional as Christopher. I didn't want to watch anymore.

"I'm tired, man; can we finish another time?"

"Sure," Finn said. "That's okay."

I left, remembering how the next day was Thursday.

I still have to write the sentence.

Pressure persisting.

* * *

When home, I said goodnight to my dad and went straight to my bedroom. With a calculation of my night and morning, I only had four hours to think of the sentence.

That is…depending on how much I sleep.

I had many questions about the movie and Chris.

What was the main character looking for? Why couldn't he embrace both the beauty of Earth and humankind? Why did I need to see this movie to figure out the sentence?

With so many intense thoughts, the night flashed by. Before I drew any conclusion, it was morning, and the house was empty.

In hasty motions, I prepared for Humanities. I showered. I dressed. I didn't eat breakfast because I wasn't hungry, and the deadline for the sentence was too soon.

Time is ticking.

I opened my blue folder and pulled out the paragraph. I carefully read every word, contemplating their significance.

How do our bodily functions consume the world and morph different perspectives? What does it look like to spend our limited time with everyone-and-everything? Is it possible to teach love in all that exists?

I needed more time for the sentence, having the urge to skip class. However, I didn't want to miss an opportunity to hear from the professor.

Maybe he'll provide the info I need to succeed.

* * *

The spring morning was lively. On my drive to campus, the temperate sun heated the inside of my dingy car. From the outside, I was directed by green signs, noticing how the bright blue sky protected me. Blackbirds flew nearby, escorting me into mindful concentration.

I felt cozy and comfortable—a haven of consciousness. Like every bit of memory, knowledge, and connection to people, places, and things rode in the passenger seat. After parking on campus, I sat with them.

A surreal gentleness and warmth filled the air. Absorbed by silence—a few birds chirped in the near distance. Through the windows, a gold filter separated me from the outside earth. The sun brightened tall pointy trees, and the wind swirled supple leaves on grassy lawns.

I grounded my hands on the steering wheel—round sides smooth and squishy. I leaned back in the snug seat, its cushions sucking me in.

The car and I became one, and I let go of the tension.

Time paused. I drifted. The utter serenity brought me to a place where nothing existed.

A space between the known and unknown. A space where I felt I was inching closer to the silver lining of the impossible.

The presence of my perception and experience—of believing in belief—kept me in my moment, in my car. Then, a dreamlike moment passed when…

Aha!

A flash of rich, colorful understanding passed through my mind. It felt as though a graceful bliss sparked from the center of my translucent self.

The sentence is coming.

Through velvety motions, I opened my notebook to a blank page. With my sharpest pencil, I wrote Einstein's famous equation. I then etched what I believed was the peak of my insight—the apex of my consciousness.

The tip's lead, scraping against the thin parchment, vibrated my body. Each word felt transcendent—as if the world was about to change forever.

This is it. This is everything.

I won. I had my answer.

Eternal life occurs when you balance thinking and doing while feeling both.

Madness severs sanity.

* * *

I faced warning signs of a crisis. Symptoms severely impaired my function. Though I hadn't exposed myself or others to unsafe situations, I could have.

I'm challenged by the complex path my symptoms took. I'm happy to have found passion in philosophy—a field of study that contributes to our capacity to understand reality. But I'm troubled that my thoughts made me so unstable and clearly influenced my illness.

The professor witnessed my uncontrollable energy when I struggled to stop talking. My father heard my bizarre thoughts about being naked in the middle of the woods and moving the cup with my mind. With Finn, I had delusional references while watching *Into the Wild*.

No one took action to get me help.

Why?

I don't blame anyone. I hope that, someday, we teach family and friends to identify warning signs. Typically, they are the first to see them. But my friends and family were never taught. So how could they see?

I couldn't recognize the professor as a hallucination when he touched my shoulder. I failed to manage my over-analytical and racing thoughts. Not sleeping for days and skipping breakfast were behaviors growing from illness.

What if the professor viewed my thoughts as a sign of a crisis? What prevented my father from seeing how unwell I was? What could have been done if Finn saw my need for help?

Not everyone's symptoms severely impair their function. But when they do, it can be serious. With more than 5 percent of adults having serious mental illness—those who are eighteen to twenty-five have double the prevalence—we need to address this issue.

My health and wellness relied on outside forces. Unless someone intervened, the risk of an incident would increase. Soon enough, I faced a critical situation. One that was unsafe for myself and others.

Would I survive?

PROPHETIC ILLUSION

I had my answer. I couldn't believe it. I discovered the sentence summary.

Eternal life occurs when you balance thinking and doing while feeling both.

With the sentence folded in my pocket, I walked toward class. A gold filter coated the sidewalks, the lawns, and the sky. My body moved in motion with the earth.

I felt enchanted. Invincible. As if the sun and wind lifted me into the kingdom of knowledge and truth, and I was at the center of everything.

Craaank! The door startled the classroom.

All eyes looked at me as I entered. Like statues, the students froze—backs straight and heads up. The professor sat while his teaching assistant spoke—his voice as stale as the air.

The room was mundane. Far too mundane for what I had just accomplished.

No one knew…yet.

I slid my sentence to the professor and took my seat. He slowly unfolded its sharp corners—my breath clutched at each separation. His eyes then scrolled over the words.

"Wow," he whispered, loud enough for everyone to hear.

Lightning struck. The professor had the same realization I did only minutes before.

He replaced his teaching assistant, stood tall, and spoke.

"The prophecy is true," I heard him say.

I trembled.

Is it possible?

My question was instantly answered. The professor described how humanity's greatest discovery was found at that very moment. He detailed the exact location, date—March 10, 2016—and time, referring to when and where the revelation was presented to him.

"Humanity has waited an eternity for this moment," he said. "It will change the world forever."

Not once did the professor make eye contact with me. But his words jolted my mind like thunder shocking the world below.

Motionless. I couldn't believe it. I was the one.

Out of the billions of people to have lived on earth, I was the one to uncover the ultimate truth.

I am...the Prophet.

* * *

New thoughts burst into my mind with intense and interlacing visions.

Now that we have this truth, how do we bring people together around it?

The second I asked the question, the Professor began answering it. I had to write the ideas down.

"Can I have paper and a pencil?" I asked a student near me.

His eyes widened and jaw stiffened—as if he feared contact with someone exceeding the scope of reality.

"C'mon, man, hurry up," I said.

My patience was thin. Every millisecond felt critical—like the world depended on me and this moment. The student eventually gave me what I needed.

Finally.

A diagram was coming to me. I divided the paper into three parts—three different sectors for the three principles of life (shown on page 125).

The top left corner showed the truth about the formation of reality—Einstein's equation explaining how we physically exist. The bottom third showed the truth about the human experience of reality—my sentence explaining how we functionally live. The middle showed the truth about human perception of reality—a drawing explaining our understanding of life and existence. The red border along the left signified the separation of what was and what was not.

I added words and symbols in each sector to indicate their connection. A combination of all three truths led me to the back of the paper—the truth of what our life could be.

Our beings were equal in every sector and mode of the truth. But something, perhaps the unexplainable part, prevented us from achieving this harmony with each other.

However, I just uncovered the missing piece.

"My teacher taught me how to teach and feel."

Am I the one to lead humanity toward peace and prosperity?

* * *

I desperately wanted to talk with the professor, but he disappeared after class. It felt like a movie moment—the rising action occurred, and the audience needed to process it. So, I understood why he didn't want to speak with me.

Besides, I discovered the most critical truth in the universe.

What could go wrong?

I left campus, and my surroundings glowed. Houses and flowers bloomed with stark colors and shapes—symmetrical wood lines of faded paint and bushes of circular accents.

The air was tender. Like bulbs from above, trees softened the atmosphere, and the sharp cement of roads revealed their mud.

Immense vitality burrowed within me. I felt bound and free—a magnetic spirit at the center of the universe.

I was supposed to feel this way. I was the one. Now, I had to bring humanity together by sharing my theory.

The most important mission in the history of existence.

I prepped for the next steps when I arrived home. I thought about the need to change our social systems—money, technology, law, culture, and all factors influencing humans had to be considered.

But how to show the change?

On a table, I placed soda bottles with varied labels, my credit cards, and my keys in a curved line. I strategically shifted the items around, capturing a pattern of words, shapes, and colors to display the change I wanted to see.

Once I felt it was right, I wanted to show the professor. I wondered if he was ready to talk and questioned why he left so quickly after class. At some point, I determined he was setting up a meeting with world leaders.

We must connect with key stakeholders to integrate our work into global culture.

When I emailed the professor, I was stunned. He had already sent me a message—as if he was reading my mind.

"Hi, Cohen…I urge you to meet with the Dean of Disabilities…she is someone I trust," the email read.

The dean was no world leader. I didn't know why I had to see her—the word "disabilities" confused me. But I did not question the professor. Whatever he said was necessary for the mission.

The dean responded to me within minutes. We were to meet the following day.

My next step.

Alluding fallacy.

* * *

I couldn't sleep. I wanted to yet the clock ticked. I kept having visions about the creation and future of the universe.

Stars exploded. Gardens rose from the ashes. Flesh and bone grew as a flower bud opened. I fell into the sea, floating above circular-shaped critters as they propagated and scattered.

Tik tik tik tik.... The clock went on, and I felt wide awake.

Eventually, I thought sleeping was a waste of time.

For what? We could accomplish so much more if we never slept.

The next thing I knew, I shot out of my bed with a burst of enthusiasm. It was bright outside. The sun was lively. My dad left for work, and, recalling the red cup, I tried to move it with my mind again.

The cup was in the same spot as before—untouched. Staring deep into its soul, my eyes wrapped around its curvy edge and gleaming color. The innards of my mind absorbed every atom of its man-made plastic.

After a few minutes, the cup never moved—*surprise.*

I need to go smaller.

Above the cup was a green leaf attached to a fake tree. Squaring my body with it, I pierced my sight into its finest details. Several moments passed by, and it didn't move.

Smaller.

On the couch were strands of my dog's fur. The thin white lines on the black fabric caught my eye as if they were meant to. Not only were they weightless and tiny, but they came from Meesha.

I sat in my spot on the couch, aligning my arms and legs. I placed a sliver strand of hair between me and moved my face inches near it. Fixing my eyes and remaining motionless, I thought of Meesha and our shared memories.

Playing fetch in the backyard. Going for walks. The more I deepened my gaze, the more my world lifted, and my peripheral vision faded.

Eventually, my breath disappeared. My body numbed. My thoughts dissipated.

This was the moment. I felt it.

Ahhh! I forced an inner thrust and bent one end of the hair inward.

Unlike how air could blow an object, the hair moved with the space it occupied.

I did it.

I leaped off the couch. I threw my hands up. I discovered what no one else had—again.

I'm gaining power.

* * *

My drive to the dean proved I was on the right path. By following signs from the universe, I achieved maximum efficiency.

I slowed down behind red cars. Red indicated danger. Blue cars meant I could pass if the speed limit permitted. White cars meant I could drive with it however I wanted. If I came across a silver car, I'd have to go by it as fast as possible.

My speedometer would bridge one hundred miles per hour. I had no fear. The universe's protection was the ultimate protection.

I reached campus in record time. I didn't know where the dean's office was but believed the signs would show me. Like a maze, I had to follow the pattern of things to make the meeting on time—late or early felt like a failure.

I frantically walked around campus, regretting my choice of sandals and jeans as they tripped me up. My posture was droopy—like my body couldn't keep up with my mind.

"You know where the Dean of Disabilities office is?" I asked a random dude.

He looked at me as if I was crazy.

The clock ticked closer to the hour, and tension swelled in my mind. I then saw blue signs on red brick buildings. Their white lettering felt secure.

I learned the office number, followed the coordinated paths, and arrived at the right spot at the right time.

The precise time.

* * *

The dean was an older woman. Her thin hair and saggy cheeks lacked color, but her grandma-like presence was warm.

Before she could introduce herself, I raved about my theory. Word after word, I paced back and forth in the free space of her small office.

"There must be more about the connection between our mind and body," I said. "Maybe it's another part of the brain—the unexplainable part."

I kicked off my sandals, wanting my body closer to earth. I pulled out a bright orange clementine from my sweater pocket.

"Do you want this delightful gift from our planet?" I asked.

She didn't accept the clementine.

"Please sit," she said.

The firmness in her voice made me listen. During my slight pause to sit, I felt someone watching us.

"Is the professor here?" I asked.

It made sense if he is. He had to observe the prophet without interruption.

"He's on vacation in another country."

I felt betrayed at first. But I recalled his meeting with world leaders.

That's exactly what he should be doing.

"How do you feel?" she asked.

My head perked.

"I'm on top of the world! Watch what I can do."

I pulled a white coffee filter from my jeans and put it on the table between us. It was a light, neutral item, and I loved coffee.

For less than a minute, I stared. It didn't move.

"Let's forget about that," she said, tossing it in the garbage. "Why are you here?"

"The professor…the theory…I discovered this sentence…"

Everything was happening so quickly. I couldn't be still.

"What do I do?" I asked.

"Go home," she said, placing her palms on the table.

"Go home, and do what? Relax on my spot on the couch? Play with my dog?"

"Yes," she replied.

Going home and relaxing is the next step.

Wishful thinking.

* * *

I was bound by the direction of the dean—as if she spoke Universal Law.

Perhaps the professor is at my house with the world leaders. Or, maybe, he and the dean were preparing something and needed more time.

I drove home the same way when going to campus. Weaving through traffic, I envisioned traveling the world to spread my word. My hope of improving humanity grew more vivid with each second.

All I have to do is follow the signs of the universe.

I did what the dean said—played with Meesha and sat in my spot on the couch. To relax, I inhaled a deep breath.

Ding ding ding. A new idea rang in my head.

On a blank page in my notebook, I wrote "5 = 3. "5 = 3." Five equaled three because they were each one oddly shaped line.

I wrote more equations. "5 = 6," "2 = 1," and so on. However, "3 ≠ 4" if you write four with two lines.

Thump. Thump. Thump. Thundering knocks roared through the house, and my heart skipped a beat.

Professor?

I sprinted to the front door. Opening it, I saw a man in a gray police uniform.

"Did the professor send you?" I asked. "Are you a police officer?"

"Ummm…no, and yes, I am a police officer."

But I assumed he was undercover for the professor.

Okay, "officer."

In hasty motions, I let the man into my home and rambled about my theory. I explained my math equations. I told him my sentence. He looked bewildered the entire time.

Does he not understand? Are my words not making him see the truth?

"If everyone saw the world like me, we'd all live happily," I said.

"But not everyone will believe what you believe," he said.

His challenge made me question myself. Suddenly, I was the bewildered one.

Am I just believing in something?

I started to feel like I was wasting my time and wanted to see the professor. I walked toward my car, and the man followed. When I saw his car blocking mine, I grew agitated.

"I need to see the professor," I said. "Please, let me go."

"Just wait here for a moment," he responded.

The man called someone. I patiently stood in the driveway—arms crossed, face down. A second later, my head perked.

Maybe he's talking to the professor…

He ended his call and walked to me.

"Can I have you come with me?"

I squinted, feeling uncertain.

"The professor would want you to do this," he added.

Something about his demeanor—his calm voice, soft smile—helped me believe him.

"Umm…okay," I said.

He put my wrists together, wrapping handcuffs around them. I felt like I had done something wrong.

"These are for your safety," he said. "Please trust me."

Since it was for the professor, I felt like I had to trust him. Then I connected the dots. The silver, circular edges were a sign from the universe. I was good to go.

Once settled in his car, we drove off.

We must be going to see the professor.

* * *

I kept my eyes closed for the entire drive. Anytime I opened them, the car aggressively shook. Clearly, I had to preserve the anonymity of the prophet's journey.

I didn't want to get in an accident and fail the mission. So, I scrunched my eyeballs, gripped my hands, and let my mind wander.

Screeech! The car stopped.

I opened my eyes—blinded by the scorching sun. I stood up; my legs feeling rickety. I didn't know where we were. But the man led me into a large, brick building.

As glass doors opened at my will, Clorox shot up my nose. White painted the floors and walls. Dozens of people paced around in white clothes.

We gotta…ring ring…bomp….bomp… Chatter, alarms, and beeps stuffed my ear pit.

Everything felt chaotic. Yet white indicated neutrality. I then saw several blue and yellow items.

Bins. Wall plugs. Signs.

I'm supposed to be here.

The man instructed me to lie in a bed squared off by a white tapestry. He removed the shiny rings and spoke to someone nearby.

I felt at ease with my wrists tension free. I laid back ready to rest when suddenly, a woman appeared.

"How did you…?" she began asking.

Stop it! Now…wha…doing wha…no…gro…elp? Loud voices cut her off.

"How did you get here?" she asked again, raising her voice.

"You take a left. Then a quick right. After a quarter-mile, you take another right..." I said, picturing a five-mile route I loved to run.

I pointed my fingers in the directions I mentioned, but she wasn't pleased. She rolled her eyes.

"Have you been sleeping lately?"

I brought up my idea of not sleeping because it was less productive.

"In fact, rather than circumcisions when born, we should remove our eyelids."

The woman's face evolved from irritation to disgust.

Wait, that doesn't make sense?

Soon after, a man in a long white coat strolled into the fabricated room.

"Comment te sens-tu?" he asked.

Hahaha! My mouth cackled.

"Really?"

I took years of French yet couldn't understand any of it. His words sounded important though. So, just like when I listened to the Hurdy-gurdy, I honed in on each sound of his voice.

"*À quand remonte la*...st time you slept?"

Like magic, his words morphed into English.

"Oh...I get it. You just have an accent."

"Good job, Cohen," he responded, smiling with me.

Oh my god, what is that?!

I felt a sharp, cold object suddenly touch my leg. I turned to see the woman wiping a cloth on me. She then grabbed a large, pointy needle off a table nearby.

"What are you doing to me?" I shrieked.

I began to leap off the bed. However, two people I didn't see grabbed my shoulders and forced me back.

"We're putting something inside you to help you," she said.

"Something in me! Why?"

I fought back, but the others overpowered me. The pinch of the needle penetrated my leg. As she pulled out, a cold bubble formed underneath my skin. It felt refreshing.

"Oh…it's water," I stated. "That makes sense."

Water was precisely what I needed in my bloodstream. The universe wanted its earthly purity running through my veins.

I must now have the ability to share my truth.

A minute later, the room went dark and silent. Black faded from the periphery of my vision. Those around me disappeared.

Like being shot in slow motion, my mind and body dissolved into itself, and I felt like I was moving on to something greater. Perhaps Heaven or a state of nothing.

Wherever a being goes when it is no longer a thing.

Mystifying deceit.

* * *

People, or myself, could have gotten hurt. A car accident. A sign to jump off a cliff. Thankfully, the professor connected me with the dean, and she contacted the police, who took me to the emergency room.

I'm grateful for everyone who supported me in getting immediate help. Although intervention could've happened earlier, when it did, the system worked. It terrifies me to know what could've happened. Especially when I hear about lethal responses to mental illness such as with Jordan Neely.

Jordan, who had a cycle of mental health crises, arrests, and hospitalizations, was killed in May 2023. He acted erratically on a Manhattan subway before being choked to death by someone else on the train.

I was acting erratically. But everyone remained calm and de-escalated the situation. As my signs revealed impaired function and an increased risk of incident, Section 9.41 of the Mental Hygiene Law allowed police to detain me.

But what if the professor never intervened? What if a cop chased me when speeding home from the dean's office? What if the police mishandled my situation, or the 9.41 was not granted?

My distorted reality due to untreated illness terrifies me. Now that I was going to the hospital, change was possible. But I had to see how sick I was. I needed appropriate support to understand my mental health and manage it.

Hospitalization alone wouldn't save me.

SUBTLY

I opened my eyes to a dim room lit by soft, yellow lamps. Sandy shades matched the mellow ambiance. It was quiet, and I felt rested. However, I didn't know where I was.

I must have teleported.

I didn't know what time it was. I didn't know what I was doing. During my teleportation, reality felt absent—as if I existed in an uncharted place that took form beyond myself.

I sat up on the bed to see a familiar face smiling at me.

"How are you feeling?" my grandma, the only other person in the room, asked.

I wasn't sure what to say. My mind felt unplugged.

"I…mmm tired," I murmured.

A second later, I shifted in my bed and rested my eyes. I began to evaporate into the unknowing darkness when, with intense velocity, I was blinded.

Beaming bulbs flashed in an instant. Fluorescent lights dizzied my pupils. Once my sight adjusted, I found myself in a different room.

How…

Glossy marble floors. Stiff cold air. Firm, peach-colored chairs. It felt like I was in the dreadful waiting room of a doctor's office.

My mom and dad appeared. They talked amongst themselves, occasionally glancing my way. From what I overheard, they were taking me somewhere.

"Taking me where?" I said, irritated. "I'm fine."

"It's okay…it's okay…" I heard.

I couldn't follow what my parents were saying, and they didn't seem to hear me either. Space flashed forward again.

Strapped onto a bed in what looked like an ambulance, I glanced to my left. Trees and clouds darted by—fuzzy pictures of a window acting like a TV.

"Wow, you slept the entire way," a man sitting nearby said.

But I couldn't respond. I couldn't even keep my eyes open.

What the hell is happening?

* * *

Cheep cheep…cheep cheep. Crickets whistled outside a glowing, twilight window.

The moon and stars brightened enough space for me to see the room I was in.

Weird.

Empty beds were nearby—white tapestries crinkled at the wall. Dressers and nightstands looked like they hadn't been used in forever. Silent air amplified their presence.

Am I in another dimension?

One door was partially open. Its crease of amber light illuminated the pale, tiled floor of this strange place.

I looked through it to see a girl my age dancing. Her warm, beige sweater matched her smile. She tapped her body—curly brown hair bouncing to a drumbeat.

I love drums.

I wanted to tell her when she noticed me—her eyes were as curious as mine. But before I could, she disappeared.

If she can walk around, can I?

I stepped through the door. Bleached light scorched my skin. Lysol choked my nostrils. I tiptoed around—head scanning like a camera.

Closed doors lined the hallway. One area housed a table and bookcase with Candyland and Monopoly. The other had a TV, baby angel art, and cement-colored chairs.

It felt like I was in a waiting room designed to be lived in.

Weird.

I stumbled upon a woman behind a long and tall desk. She wore faint blue scrubs.

"Where am I?" I asked.

"You're in a psych ward in Olean," she said.

Olean?

I didn't know where that was.

Psych ward?

I didn't know what that meant. Other than depictions of people acting nuts—wild hair, odd body movements—I didn't understand what a psych ward really was.

I knew I wasn't crazy.

"What am I supposed to do here?"

"Relax," she said.

Okay.

I sat on a cement-colored chair. I inhaled deep breaths. I caressed my quads.

My T-shirt read Geneseo Track and Field. My sweatpants tugged at my heels. My…

Wait…what the?

These ugly, puke-yellow socks clutched my feet. Sticky white stuff gripped their bottoms.

I didn't remember putting them on.

Did I black out or something?

A hospitalized trance.

* * *

One by one, the hallway doors opened. One by one, people gathered around.

A lanky man with black stubble on his face—maybe early thirties—walked directly to the baby angel art.

"Mary, it's me. Jesus. Jesus knows," he said, hands in prayer.

A hefty man wearing glasses—maybe my age—sat nearby. I tried making eye contact. But he quickly turned the other way.

Then, the girl who drummed appeared. My chest palpitated. On the floor, she laid out crayons and a coloring book.

I wanted to talk to her, but she looked focused. So, I tried again with the hefty man. This time, our eyes met.

"I'm Cohen. Who are you?"

"Will," he said.

I recalled *Good Will Hunting*. A film where a janitor solves a math equation that changes the world.

Maybe I have a reason to meet Will.

"Why are you here?" I asked.

"Suicidal thoughts. But I'm feeling better."

He was chatty once the ice was broken. We talked about video games and movies. He described his love for cooking and how the food here sucked.

The girl who drummed kept glancing our way like she wanted to join the conversation.

"Can we color with you?" I asked.

"Sure!" she said.

Will wasn't interested. But I was quick to sit with her.

"What image do you want?" she asked, handing me a book with psychedelic illustrations.

I ripped out a page that outlined a human meditating at a square's center and planned my scheme. Four separate sectors for four different crayons. The colors, well…they had to mean something.

AHHHHH! A blood-curdling scream pierced my eardrums.

At first, I thought someone was being tortured. When I twisted my back to see the sound, I didn't seem far off.

On the ground, an elderly woman in flowery sleepwear was screaming at the ceiling. Two people in scrubs were dragging her into a room.

"She just needs a picture of a fireplace," the girl who drummed said. "Then she'll no longer be cold."

I imagined a shrunken fire squared in a frame—brown tones and orange flames centering my eyes.

She's right. It'd make me think of being warm.

I began realigning my shoulders, ready to color, when I saw a bald man with a thick goatee. He stood at the tall desk, thrusting his fists up and down.

"I will not take it," he yelled at a lady in scrubs. "Medication is from the devil!"

What's happening here?

I would've never assumed medication was from the devil. Although the man with the goatee seemed adamant about not taking the pill, he eventually did.

Plot twist.

I finished coloring the four corners with green, red, yellow, and blue. The outline of a human mediating remained colorless. My idea was that, for far too long, society thwarted people's needs due to greed, anger, and other selfish qualities. The silhouette represented our need to be absent from them—the colors—to achieve peace.

Once finished, I shared it with the girl who drummed.

"Color theory, you got it," she nodded.

Maybe I'm onto something.

* * *

The girl who drummed explained how she landed in the psych ward. She was fighting her mom and threatened to kill her.

"I'd never actually hurt her though. I love her," she emphasized. "I was just mad."

I didn't know about their relationship. I didn't know about her home life. But I understood how easy it is to say certain words when angry. I was never pleasant when I fought with my parents.

"Damn…thanks for sharing," I said. "I'm sorry you have to be here."

"What about you?" She asked.

Huh…

I didn't know the exact answer to that.

"Ummm…I saw the world differently. The professor noticed something in me. Color theory…."

"Is Cohen Miles-Rath here?" a sudden voice asked, towering over the room.

I was shocked someone knew me. I had only told Will my name.

I stood up and raised my hand. A man in a white coat glared at me.

"Follow me, please."

I was nervous. I didn't know what was going to happen.

We sat in an empty bedroom, and he asked me who I was, how I arrived at the ward, and what I felt. I had no idea who he was, yet he wanted to know a lot about me.

I stayed quiet.

"I'm a psychiatrist, you know."

"Okay," I said.

"And you had a psychotic break."

Okay...

Sensing my confusion, he drew two cups on a notebook. He added lines to indicate where the liquid stopped. One line was lower than the other.

"This cup is stable," he said, pointing to the one with the lower line. "But yours became too full and spilled over."

He added more lines to the other cup to show the overflow.

"What we do here is to prevent your cup from becoming too full again."

"But I feel fine," I said.

"You acted bizarre," he said.

"But I am not bizarre now."

Silence.

He brought up medication. I remembered the man with the goatee.

"I don't want meds. I just wanna go home," I said.

"If you want to leave, you must take the medication."

Silence.

Tension swelled in my head. Ticks of annoyance and discomfort. I didn't want to argue with this man. I didn't want to feel this way. So, I said what he wanted to hear.

"I'll take the meds."

* * *

The girl who drummed had left the common area, but Will remained. As I sat nearby, he made a gun with his hand and pointed it at the lanky man who was still talking to the baby angel art. The second he saw me, he dropped his arms as though I caught him doing something wrong.

"He's kind of loud, isn't he?" I said with a smile.

He smiled back.

Who wouldn't be annoyed by someone talking gibberish all morning?

I was curious about the lanky man. His words were unique and odd. Although scrambled initially, the more I tuned in, the more I wanted to know.

I started approaching him when the girl who drummed appeared. She asked Will and me to play a board game.

Can't say no to that.

For the rest of the day, we hung out. We ate lunch and dinner together—Will was right, the food sucked. In the evening, we huddled around the TV, watching *Gone with the Wind* and the news.

I began to appreciate the offbeat world I was in. Those behind the tall desk didn't sit with us. They stood over us. Yet we did what we wanted, even if it was talking to wall art.

I was reminded of one of my favorite mental bands System of a Down. Their melodies, often representing anarchy and unrest, matched what I was feeling.

"What disorder?" I said under my breath. "What disorder!"

I wanted to capture these feelings in my own way. So, I began composing a fictional story of life in a psychiatric ward. To be told through a mixture of flashbacks and real time, I would base the characters on my experience.

The main group—the lanky man, the man with the goatee, the girl who drummed, Will, and the distant elderly woman—were sent to the hospital against their will. Society had shunned them for something out of their control.

The group hoped to return to the outside world. But the antagonists—staff and society—wouldn't let them, using fear and shame for control. The plot would thicken as they didn't expect a hero—the main character represented by myself—to form a friendship among the group. A friendship that had been inconceivable to society.

Led by the hero, the group would explore each character's journey to the ward. We'd see their past and personalities form. We'd gain empathy with understanding.

The hero would then craft a concept—an image of a silhouette perhaps—to set them free. Not physically free, but metaphorically breaking the shackles society put them in.

In the end, the group would forgive their desire to leave because they found something no one could take from them. A realization that they only needed acceptance from themselves.

I turned my idea into an outline on paper and carefully stored it near my bed.

Maybe that will be the movie I write.

* * *

Before bedtime, a nurse requested me at the tall desk. She handed me a small cup with a tiny white pill in it. I remembered my meeting with the psychiatrist and took the medication as promised.

I walked toward my room when I noticed the lanky man still in the common area. This time, he was talking to the TV. With no one else around, I took my chance to speak with him.

"What's your name?" I asked.

"You know Jesus? I know Mary. She came to me. Joseph too. They know me," he rambled. "See, things happen in three. One. Two. Three. That's the secret."

In the news tonight, a man was arrested for.... Voices on the TV instantly snagged his attention.

"See! They're watching. Look," he added, pointing to the TV.

The more he spoke, the more I realized I had to listen to his words rather than ask questions. So I did.

I patiently stood. I kept eye contact. I focused on his words of God, numbers, and patterns.

Something in the way he spoke made me feel like he was trying to figure something out. Something important.

Has he been in my mind before?

Suddenly, I had an idea.

"What do you think of eternal life?" I asked.

For the first time, he went dead silent—eyes fixed on mine.

"What about this sentence? Eternal life occurs when you balance thinking and doing while feeling both."

His eyes widened. The corners of his lips lifted.

"You write scripture?"

Before I could respond, he zoomed away and returned with a Holy Bible.

"Can you write that here?"

He opened it to the first blank page. I grabbed a green marker and wrote in my best handwriting. As I gave it back, he reached out to shake my hand.

"My name's Arthur. A. R. for short."

Finally.

I was onto something.

Stimulating symptoms.

* * *

Throughout the following days, I began sharing the sentence with everyone. The girl who drummed. The therapists, counselors, or whoever it was prying at my mind. No one reacted much until I met with one doctor.

I had yet to see this man. He looked older than the others and wore a tie under his coat.

"How are you feeling?" he asked—his strong accent amplifying his confidence.

Stay cool. Stay cool…

I didn't want to say how annoyed I was. I had been ready to go home for several days.

"Relaxed," I said.

"You're taking medication, correct?"

"Yes, every night."

We sat through a long pause until his eyes started to glint.

"What you create is genius," he said with a smile.

If I'm some genius, why do I have to be here?

I shrugged my shoulders. I didn't want to risk not being able to leave.

"How much longer do I have to stay here?" I asked.

"A minimum of five days. Depends on your progress."

Okay…good news.

I was on my fourth day and was doing good.

Why keep me?

Later that night, it was confirmed. My parents were picking me up the following afternoon.

* * *

I was excited. I wanted to get back to my routine of work and college. I wanted to see family and friends—some of whom had called me.

Finn said we could play a show as soon as I returned. My siblings Cody and Lindsay said I would be okay—that I didn't need to be in the hospital. My parents believed I was good too.

Everyone thought I was fine.

Because I am...right?

I thought about weed. Five days was a long time not to smoke. I told others about my desire. Surprisingly, the girl who drummed insisted I didn't.

"It's not good for you," she said.

It isn't? Really?

When the therapists said the same thing, I wanted to smoke more.

Who the hell are they to tell me what to do?

* * *

The first thing I did before my parents picked me up was acquire a manilla envelope. I had to secure my work, including the screenplay outline and the psychedelic drawing I colored.

As I put my work into the envelope, I saw a pattern—a way to tell a story through the sequence of creases. For several minutes, I folded the sheets in coordination with their colors and words. I felt a more profound meaning with them—as if my story, experience, and desire to share were all connected.

Fascinating.

Before my final lunch there, a nurse approached me.

She looked at those in the common area, and said, "You're the only one who isn't crazy here, aren't you?"

I was taken aback—annoyed and pissed off.

My friends aren't crazy.

I sat in the dining hall with the girl who drummed. In the corner, the elderly woman talked to herself with the occasional, unforeseen shriek. The man with the goatee, eating a meaty sandwich, gritted his teeth at her.

"I pray y'all don't end up like that," he said, looking at me and the girl who drummed.

I was caught off-guard. We barely spoke, and I didn't expect compassion from him.

Although his comment was brief, I felt supported. I felt grateful for him and all the peers I met in the hospital. They helped me see. They helped me realize how genuine kindness could come from anyone—no matter their story.

They were the reason I was there.

Resurrected fiction.

* * *

I didn't understand why I went to the hospital. I didn't want to go and only accepted medication to leave. I didn't trust anyone but my peers. I did not want help because I couldn't see I was unwell.

Whether I liked it or not, I had to go. With Section 9.39 of the Mental Hygiene Law, emergency room doctors could admit me because they believed I posed a substantial risk of physical harm to myself and others.

Although I wish systems of support did more to encourage voluntary hospitalizations, I now see the importance of being forced to go. Something worse could've happened. But I'm concerned about the treatment team's failure to make me realize I was unwell. Knowing what could've been prevented, I wish these moments of significant intervention were effective.

Doctors used Ambien to sedate me before the transition. After sleeping, the severity of signs and symptoms decreased. However, they didn't go away. It was bizarre to see a pattern when folding my work into the manilla envelope. When sharing the sentence with A. R., I felt like I was onto something—a resemblance to my symptoms before.

I don't think the treatment team knew enough about my experience to fully understand. I struggled to explain, and I didn't trust them. Progress notes capture their observations.

> *He states that because he was thinking strange, he was behaving strange, and he was feeling strange. He states that he has gained perspective and now plans to put these grand thoughts into the format of a paper and utilize it for school versus getting wrapped up in it the way that he was.*

The notes don't show I understood the illness or embraced treatment. To me, I simply had a weird experience and overcame it. To them, medication was the answer.

> *A twenty-two-year-old male with no psychiatric history was admitted to the hospital post a psychosis episode, which has subsequently resolved via the use of Risperdal.*

Unlike many physical illnesses, mental illness cannot be solved by medication alone. Even with wrap-around services, support would not be as effective if I couldn't see how unwell I was or communicate my symptoms.

I don't blame the treatment team. But to think meds are the answer is naive and over-simplistic, and the harm that does angers me. However, clinicians I've let read these progress notes say they would have done the same.

So then what is it?

Our entire mental health approach struggles to foster insight, growth, and hope. It's even more sad when you consider the history of treatment.

Before the late 1900s, people were isolated in asylums, strapped to beds, or forced to wear straightjackets. Through lobotomies, people's brains were scraped with a metal tool that looked like scissors. Some of these ineffective practices still occur in the world.

Although we've improved mental health care, we have a long way to go. Though barbaric forms of coercive treatment are rare today, we still look for simple solutions—*just take these pills*—to complex problems.

What if I went through a less frightening method of urgent care—would have I been more likely to listen to the doctors? What if, instead of forced medication, treatment relied on support from loved ones, peers, and providers who engaged in a process of change rather than an immediate fix? What if I had learned about mental health and understood I was unwell—would have I accepted help?

My mental health needs weren't adequately addressed. My wellness depended on the continuing support I would or would not receive and my ability or inability to manage my mental health.

Would I remain stable?

MISTAKEN FREEDOM

I was in the hospital during spring break from college. I didn't have to miss class or explain why I was absent. I could get back to my life as if nothing happened.

I attended Humanities and French. I worked at Fusion. I freshened up my resume and researched careers at Teach for America and the Peace Corps. Although my ideas with screenplay writing and the theory dissipated, remnants of my confinement lingered.

"You have to see an outpatient therapist once a month," a social worker at the hospital said, scheduling the first session before I left.

I didn't want to go. Why would I want to go?

I am fine. I am fine. I am fine.

"It's great you're in school and work," the therapist said. "Maybe we can look at your resume next time you're in."

When she asked about medication, I was honest.

"I stopped taking them. I think I'm fine. I don't like the idea of meds."

My dad had agreed meds were not a good idea. He worried about the side effects. And my anger was increasing.

Maybe a side effect. Maybe an excuse.

"I strongly encourage you to take them," she said. "Especially since you just left a psychiatric center."

I knew she couldn't understand my experience, however. I couldn't even explain it.

"It was a fluke," I said.

I told her the sentence, using it to describe my idea of pursuing philosophy.

"Maybe I could get a master's instead of starting work."

"If that's something you want to study, it could be a good idea," she said.

I knew I was onto something.

* * *

I smoked weed daily, getting high before work and Humanities again. The professor never spoke about the sentence or the dean. We engaged in small talk—student and teacher—and that was it.

My family didn't address my hospitalization either. My brothers, sisters, and parents pretended nothing had happened. Even my friends did the same.

As the days passed, the entire experience felt less real—like a temporary moment of a mystifying dream. I was happy to have it swept under the rug.

I wasn't crazy.

But one night, I was at Finn's house talking to his mom.

"I was there for like five days…not sure why," I said. "The doctors mentioned schizophrenia or something, but I have nothing to worry about. I feel good."

"Schizophrenia is serious," she said, expressing concern before I walked off with Finn.

For a moment, I wondered if I should learn more about schizophrenia. I had only heard of it a handful of times in my life.

What is it, and why was it brought up?

"Just let all that shit go," Finn said as we readied our instruments and played by the campfire. "Weed put you in the wrong mind."

I listened to him. I let it all go. But I didn't listen to him entirely. I had been high the entire time at his house.

Nothing will go wrong again.

* * *

Finn and I played a concert at a local bar. I had looked forward to my first opportunity to go out since the hospital. He invited me to stay at his friend's, so I was able to exploit the bar.

Drink after drink. Smoke after smoke. The night morphed into a blurry mess.

The morning after, a throbbing headache prevented me from continuing to sleep. I didn't remember getting to the house—or most of the night. But when I smoked a bowl, I felt better.

All is good.

The house was quiet and peaceful. Since it was before 8:00 a.m., I was the only one awake. Always prepared to do homework, I settled in the dining room and opened my backpack. When grabbing Sigmund Freud's *Civilization and Its Discontents*—a required reading for Humanities—I saw my blue folder wedged between binders and books.

How could I forget about that?

I pulled out the folder and set it aside. Something about it felt cryptic.

Should I open it?

I let Freud's book distract me. My assignment was to read and write a paper. Within a few minutes, I read about the "oceanic feeling." The concept sounded as beautiful as its definition.

"It is a feeling which he would like to call a sensation of 'eternity,'" Freud wrote. "A feeling as of something limitless, unbounded—as it were, 'oceanic.'"

Interesting...very interesting.

I stopped working on the paper. I opened my blue folder. I read its contents and used Freud's work to examine mine.

"I cannot discover this 'oceanic' feeling in myself," he continued to say. "It is not easy to deal scientifically with feelings."

He referred to his psychoanalytic theory—the framework of feelings associated with the ego. He connected the concept with religious sentiments, mentioning how that attitude stems from infantile helplessness.

In the end, Freud argued the concept's lack of tangible qualities and chalked it up to a form of idealistic perception.

"Let him rejoice who breathes up here in the roseate light!" he quoted German poet Friedrich Schiller.

New ideas swarmed into my mind. I inscribed words, letters, and scribbles onto clean, white paper.

If one cannot find fact in feeling, then what is fact?

Philosophical thought sparked within me once again. An electric force evoking the veins inside my skull.

Why did I stop pursuing my theory? Why did I give up?

A stranger entered the dining room. He looked out the window, pushing its drapes aside. His long brown hair, beard, and robe glistened in the fresh sunlight.

I assumed he was a house resident, but something felt different.

"What are you working on?" he asked.

"That's a loaded question," I said, handing him the sheets from my folder. "I believe Freud has a fault in his theory about how our minds work. He's missing something."

He shuffled through my papers.

"Maybe you've figured it out," he said, smiling.

Moments later, Finn woke up. As we gathered ourselves to leave, the man disappeared. I stowed my work in my backpack and snuck a few hits from my bowl.

What's next?

* * *

It had been three weeks since I left the hospital—time that separated me from my mission. But I felt restored—recognizable energy crescendoing with every thought.

What was it with that man in the dining room?

I recalled the manilla envelope from the hospital.

Where did that go? I need my next steps.

I frantically searched my house. Sadly, I couldn't find it.

Aha!

It was Jesus in the dining room.

He came to put me on the right path.

I walked into Humanities with a familiar anticipation. As usual, the classroom felt bleak. The students looked like assembly line machines—conformed to a reality they couldn't break.

"Are we ready to begin the online exam?" said the professor at the exact moment I sat.

Like crash cymbals, paranoia collided my stomach and mind. I feared not having my laptop. But when I opened my backpack, it was in the right place.

The precise place.

I turned on my computer, eager to discover a clue in the exam. However, a forced update intensified my anxiety.

Is something working against me?

"Don't let the computer Gods stop you," I heard the professor say to a student.

Isn't the Universe on my side?

Eventually, I accessed the exam and answered most of it with nonsense. Only one question felt essential to the mission. A question examining science and religion and if both could be true.

I immediately thought of the biblical story of Adam and Eve in the Garden of Eden. I didn't want to explore how the garden came into existence. Any explanation—religious or scientific—felt irrelevant. I cared more about what it meant for beings to live among one another and all other things.

So, I removed the religious application, noted natural science could describe substances and their functions, and examined the story through a social scientific lens.

> *Two humans appear in a garden. They know what they see—a sharp red circle hanging on a pointy, soft brown line. The unique, motionless red intrigues them. When they hear a thing unknown—a hissing nearby—they grab the red to know more.*

Everything in the story was based on causes and effects. Subjects capable could interpret the goodness or badness of grabbing the apple. Fundamentally, however, what occurred was the result of things interacting because they were in each other's presence.

When interpreting anything, interaction fundamentals are key. Not assumed morals or existence explanations.

Easy.

* * *

I had to work at Fusion after class. My mind and body automatically adjusted to the different environment.

My first duty was to slice avocados. I intently rubbed their round, slightly rough edges. I pictured the bright green mush existing beneath their dark green skin.

No need to peel to see the bright green. Once I did though, I saw exactly what I imagined.

I'm getting better at balancing my thinking and doing.

"Isn't this avocado amazing?" I said to a nearby coworker. "The way it feels and what it does for us."

No words. Just a weird look before she hurried off somewhere else.

I continued appreciating the world around me. It felt like I didn't have to seek the answers anymore because the truth was embedded in me.

All I have to do is get people to feel what I feel.

The first step in achieving my goal was to connect with others. The second step was to interact in a way that shifted their thinking, doing, and feeling toward the balance.

I put my theory into practice while serving food. Hungry humans lined up at my station, craving the sandwich I made. I smiled at all of them, thinking how amazing it felt to feed the great people of my college.

When a person ordered, I embraced their presence.

"I'd like the pork belly please...."

Their squishy cheeks emulated my squeezing of the meat with tongs. A smile from my own cheeks connected us to this centerfold. As though I absorbed every element of our interaction, my being's entirety felt devoted to this exchange.

One by one, more people ordered. One by one, I felt a deeper meaning with them, recognizing the strength of our connected community.

We were free from stress. We were free from conflict. We enjoyed the fruits of life together.

That was it.

I'm accomplishing my goal.

Ill optimism.

* * *

I passed a large church when leaving work. It had gothic architecture and big red doors—a building I usually passed without any thought. This time, however, its front sign held a message.

"Wednesday Service: 12:00 p.m."

That's tomorrow. I have to go.

Not long after seeing the sign, I had a sudden memory from work. A customer, resembling the dean, looked at me as if she knew who I was.

She knows I'm the prophet. Is the professor observing me again?

The second this question popped into my mind, I noticed every driver who passed me wore black sunglasses. They kept their heads very still and forward, avoiding eye contact.

More observers.

I welcomed the professor studying me. I wanted it to fuel my leadership. If others understood how I interacted with the world, they'd be more likely to understand what I wanted to share.

That's why the professor only engaged in small talk after the hospital. He didn't want to disrupt the process.

* * *

Continuing home, a sign told me to visit my siblings Casie and Taylor. I had arrived unannounced before, so it wasn't unusual.

I took a seat in Taylor's bedroom. He, his girlfriend, and Casie passed around a bong. When given to me, I denied it. At some point, I stopped smoking weed because I wanted to be in my natural state—unaltered by extrinsic influences.

I don't need to be high to feel one with the world.

We watched TV and talked. We laughed and smiled. I felt a balance forming in the room. An aura that made me think it was working—they were shifting into the same natural state I had been in.

I needed to capture the transfiguration.

"I want a tattoo," I said to Casie. "A sentence."

"Which one?" She asked.

I tested my words, hoping to strengthen the shift happening in her mind. But she didn't respond. She was distracted by her smartphone.

I peered over her shoulder to see what brought her out of touch with our immediate presence. The second I focused on her screen, she paused on a Facebook video where a man spoke into the camera, talking about the meaning of life.

"We are all here right now, and we need to see this," the man stated. "We have no greater meaning than what is here right now. But who will help us see this?"

Casie scrolled past the video as if she knew the clue was evident to me.

I'm the one to help them see. But how to do it with billions of people?

Social media was an idea I didn't have before. But it made sense. Technology had advanced just in time for me to reach the entire world.

I knew I had a reason to see my siblings.

I began to leave, giving hugs and saying goodbye like a typical visit. As I stepped from his bedroom and down a staircase, Taylor's voice caught my ear.

"All you have to do is follow the signs," he said. "Just follow the signs."

The universe couldn't have given me a more glaring message.

Delusion revived.

* * *

I disregarded the hospital visit. I resented the therapy session. I ignored suggestions from the treatment providers. I truly believed I was okay.

I struggle with this. Do I feel sorry for myself? Do I blame myself?

I didn't have to binge drink and smoke weed. I didn't have to obsess with the theory again. But could I alone prevent my signs and symptoms from worsening?

Can I forgive myself?

I don't know if I hallucinated the man I thought was Jesus, or if he was a resident. However, I'm confident I hallucinated the drivers in black sunglasses. I don't believe Casie and I saw the same Facebook video or that Taylor actually said to follow the signs.

Looking back, I'm not surprised by my response to treatment and the results. If I couldn't accept mental illness in the hospital, I wasn't going to accept it out of the hospital.

Opportunities for support continued to be available. But again, mental health care is and has been limited. It took the COVID-19 pandemic to make a larger push for mental health investments. The organization I now work for has received grants specific to mental health training in schools.

Universities are following suit. In 2019, almost a third of U.S. higher education institutions allocated more mental health funding as compared to 2016—the year I was in crisis.

Maybe if the professor had been trained on mental health, which often talks about the need for continuing support after a crisis, he would have followed up after my hospitalization. He could have connected me with resources, offered to be flexible with assignments, or maybe something else.

Too late though.

My family, friends, and colleagues missed the mark too. They ignored the seriousness of my hospital visit. My father was okay with me stopping my medication. Although I brought up schizophrenia to Finn's mom, we brushed it off.

What if I had more support as I transitioned from the hospital to the community, and what would that look like? What if people close to me encouraged treatment, particularly my father, the professor, or Finn—those who knew I was facing a mental health challenge? What if I understood what schizophrenia was—would I have taken it more seriously?

Two journeys were ahead of me. One in my head that put me in charge of changing the world. One driven by an illness that severely impaired my function. Both were likely to cause significant disruption in my life.

How long until another crisis struck?

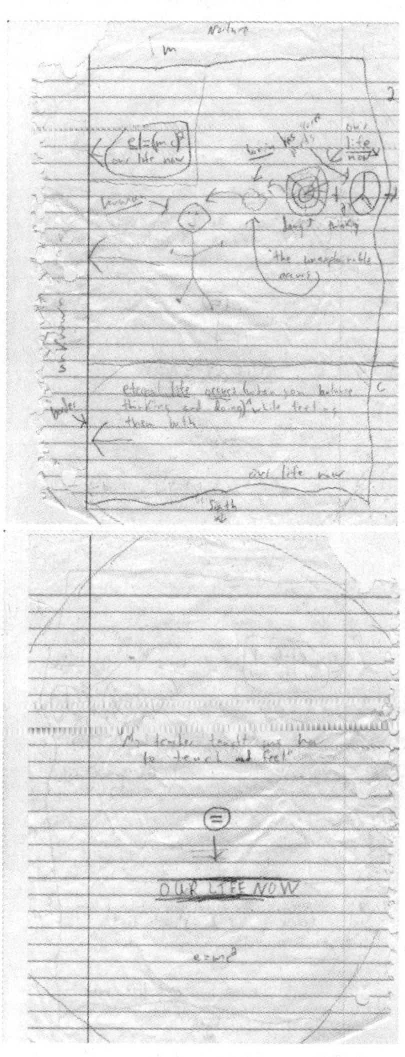

Front and back of the diagrams from Humanities class

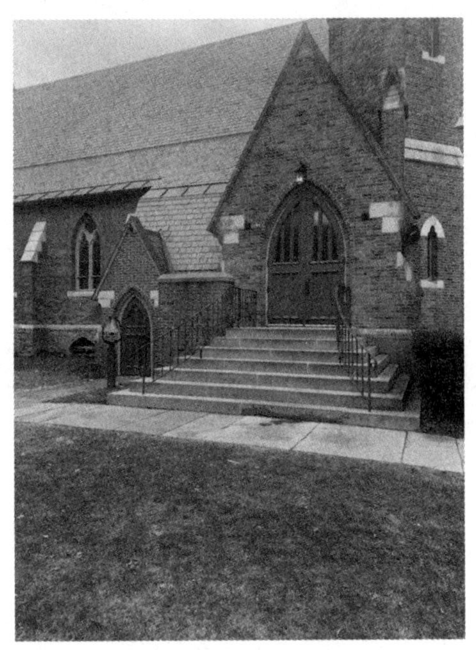

The church with the big red doors

PART III

YEARNING FANTASY

"Wednesday Service: 12:00 p.m." the church sign said. I dropped everything ten minutes before the hour. Someone agreed to cover my remaining shift at Fusion. My manager told me to wash dishes before leaving.

I scrubbed and shined every square and circular dish with speed only a person with particular balance could achieve. The manager was surprised at how fast I finished. But I wasn't. I was out the door.

In the blink of an eye, I stood at the big red doors. I expected to see rows of people facing a preacher. But the large hall was dark and empty. One person played piano in the back corner.

Why am I here?

I strolled down the center aisle, smooth piano notes charting my steps. Like the childhood game hopscotch, I bounced over the floor's patterned lines. Its geometric abstraction felt like a guide on how to passionately move with calculated rhythm.

At the altar's exact center, I looked up, mesmerized by the building's round vault and knife-like pinnacles. Stained glass windows illuminated the dim hall with enough color for me to feel safe—comfortable that I was in the right space.

*Humm...ahh...*I paused.

The lively air grounded me. My feet cemented to the floor. My shoulders solidly squared.

Seized by an immersion of sacredness, my mind…my body…

They're here…I am here…I am him….

My praying hands flowed with my heart's chest—a spiritual entwinement strengthening as my senses amplified, and my consciousness ascended.

Up and up and up…my body rose, and my mind diffused. Out and out and out…a brush of cool air coursed through my presence.

Not a moment later and…strike! Divinity entranced my being—as if God's hand reached out and touched my soul.

Similar to when I wrote the sentence, everything I had known—everything I was searching for—was coming together. But this time, just like the church's aspiring patterns and shapes, visions of humanity's future and what had to be done decorated my being.

I was a blank slate colored by an ideal world. I was a being of eternal transcendence.

I am going to change humanity forever.

I was going to change forever.

* * *

I visited the pianist before leaving.

"Thank you for playing," I said. "You're amazing."

"Just doing a little practice," he said.

I learned his name. He was Finn's uncle.

A personal connection helped create my transformation.

That made sense.

"Finn's a great musician, too," I said.

"He sure is."

I left the church, and the sunny sky awakened my eyes. Unlike the day I discovered the sentence, I felt calmer—like my ability to manage the truth was more durable.

I followed pink arrows painted on the road's edge. They took me to a restaurant called the Big Tree Inn. I smelled food wafting from the building—hunger weighed on my stomach. I couldn't recall the last time I ate.

"Can I get a meal?" I asked the lady at the front desk.

"Of course," she said, grabbing a menu.

I checked to see if I had my wallet. I didn't.

"Do I have to pay?"

She looked suspicious.

"I'm sorry…we don't give food out for free."

Does she not know I'm the prophet?

I was disappointed. I served food all morning, but no one would serve me. So, I left and drove home. When I saw my dad prepping dinner, it made sense.

I'm meant to eat with him.

We watched TV while eating—the usual. But this time, I was overwhelmed by the combination of colors, patterns, and sounds. Ideas of space, time, and human connection were woven into every film beat, coordinating my thoughts as if I were not alone.

I was unsure of my next step until I saw two people marrying. Together, the two families smiled and hugged. The wedding looked lavish—perfect people on a perfect day.

Two profoundly vivid and circular gold rings appeared on the screen.

I must marry Carrie.

* * *

Carrie, my ex-girlfriend, was on my mind throughout the next day. Marriage was essential for the mission.

But when would it happen?

I arrived at Humanities. While the professor lectured, he gave subtle hints that my next sign was elsewhere.

Duh…the teacher already taught me how to teach.

I rushed out of the classroom. Signs led me to Fusion.

I had yet to serve people food.

I had no shift, but they welcomed my help. So, once again, I served the great people of SUNY Geneseo. That was until the next sign appeared.

"She is your love, she is your love," I heard a song sing in the restaurant. "Now go on and marry her, marry her, marry her."

Destiny is calling.

Without fear or doubt, I texted Carrie, "Will you marry me?"

Waiting for her response, every second felt slower—my heartbeat increasing.

What if she says no?

Minutes passed, and she had yet to respond. So, I abandoned work and called her. She answered.

"You have to marry me," I said. "You have to."

"We're not getting married," she said. "I have to go."

I heard what I wanted to hear. She had to go because she was already at the church.

We're getting married right then and there.

I ran up the campus hill toward the big red doors. I expected to see the hall lit up with people waiting for me. But once I opened them, it was dark and deserted.

My heart sank.

How could this be?

I paced up and down the middle aisle, hopping over the patterned lines as I did the day before. I called Carrie again, expressing my love and apologizing for my mistakes.

She cried, telling me to move on.

"Are you okay, Cohen?" she asked.

"Of course I'm okay. Never been better."

I heard someone knock on her bedroom door. As she let them in, they whispered something I couldn't understand.

"I have to go," she said, quickly hanging up.

I was bewildered. But I then realized the secret whisperer must've been someone sent by the professor.

She just found out I'm the prophet.

At the exit of the church, I stumbled upon a book surrounded by red candles. I opened it and read its prompt.

"Leave your prayer here to be read in the next service."

I was a child the last time I prayed, repeating the same lines before sleep.

I pray I succeed after high school. I pray my family will become happier. I pray everyone in the world can live comfortably.

Although that wouldn't be my prayer, I knew what would be.

"Please, let her forgive me," I wrote, kneeling before the candles.

The feeling of lead on paper was similar to when I first wrote the sentence. Therefore, I knew it was more powerful than words on paper.

I'm the one sending a message to the universe.

* * *

I was returning to the restaurant when suddenly a girl in pink shoes ran past me. I looked at the time. Track practice was in five minutes.

Perfect.

I sensed the team's shock when they saw me in the locker room. It had been a long time. But as if nothing changed, I put on my running gear and followed them to the meeting spot.

Coach Dan, still a coach at the college, was instructing the plan for practice—an easy run. I asked if I could join the guys.

He looked surprised but welcomed me.

"If you can keep up," he said.

The run felt quick. Two miles in, I challenged the fastest runner in the group to a mid-run sprint. Bad idea—I was soon hunched over my belly, gasping for air.

The team laughed, mistaking my challenge for a joke. But I didn't care. At three miles in, I split off to run a shorter route by myself.

The final stretch was down the steep hill of campus. An outbreak of energy forced me to sprint.

I tightly turned on dirt pathways. I flew over obstacles.

Stone walls. Tree stumps. Staircase handrails.

I could be a professional parkour athlete.

When I reached the lower part of campus, I was near Coach Dan's office. I couldn't remember the last time we had a conversation. But I stormed in, glancing at the clock to see it was exactly thirty minutes since I began my run.

Everything is happening in thirty-minute increments.

The conversation with Coach Dan was a blur. We probably talked about the team and how his training had gone since the Ironman. At one point, I was munching on orange carrots from his mini-fridge.

"Mmm, these are refreshing," I said.

For the entire time, I kept my eye on the clock. When the next half hour hit, I sped out of his office and toward my car. I was ready to leave until…

I saw a Starbucks sign.

To succeed in my mission, I need influence—to be a star—and funds—to have the bucks.

* * *

I entered the cafe. It was loud and busy. Dozens of people roamed about. Yet the area felt intimate.

Charcoal walls. Chestnut tables. Thin streams of dim light.

A modern design with cozy comforts.

I was ready to pay this time. I swiped my card, grabbed my coffee, and sat.

Unlike Books & Bites, where people ignored the world's wonder, this place felt prosperous. Everyone, of all shapes and forms, looked perfectly beautiful, enjoying the space together.

Their smiles. Their glistening eyes. Their joyous speech.

What could be more marvelous?

It was working. Since I began putting my theory into practice, it must have spread throughout campus like a virus.

Mesmerized by the shifting ways of society, I withdrew from my thoughts. I brought my hands together. I slowed my breathing and embraced an overwhelming attachment to the earth.

My body oozed—fingers and toes melting like stone turning to lava.

Wooosh…wooosh…wooosh. A blissful noise rang, overpowering the shop's loudness.

I felt exceptionally associated with the sound—as if I was the only one to hear it.

But what is it?

Its intensity grew the more I sharpened my focus. Soon enough, it occurred to me.

I was hearing the earth spinning in space. Earth accepted me as one with its universe.

My prayer worked.

My illness swelled.

* * *

When I was ready to leave campus, a sign appeared once again. Someone in striking blue shoes walked up a set of stairs in the main hall. They led me to a long, empty hallway.

The walls were plastered with words, drawings, and pictures. They represented campus clubs building houses in countries with high poverty rates, supportive voices for marginalized communities, and other social justice initiatives.

I felt proud of my university. So many people wanted to help others—create a world where fewer people suffered, and those with disadvantages were supported.

Isn't that what I'm trying to do with my theory?

I arrived at the end of the hallway to find a door with red and white magnetic words. I began rearranging them, wondering how to connect with more people.

I have the truth and can share it personally. But how to efficiently do that with billions of humans worldwide?

Perhaps another sentence.

"Cohen Miles-Rath, Cohen Miles-Rath, Cohen Miles-Rath!" people chanted while I tried to discover it.

My friends, family, and team...they must be waiting for me at the stairs.

Words, words, words—pressure intensified as the task's difficulty increased, reminding me of creating the first sentence.

What is it? What is it? What if I can't do it?

The idea of failure raised the hair on my neck. So much so I had to pause to calm myself. Rather than staying in my mind, I scanned the decorated walls in search of a clue.

Boom. One word stuck out.

Fraternity.

Fraternity—the feeling of mutual support and a willingness to share—made sense.

Fraternity is the balance of thinking then doing while feeling both.

I glorified the celebration that awaited me at the stairs. Maybe I'd see Carrie.

Maybe I had needed the second sentence before we could marry.

However, when I arrived, I saw no one. No faces of friends or family. No waving or clapping. Just students on their way to class.

Who was chanting then?

It didn't matter. The idea of a new world—one where everyone felt the beautiful presence of each other and each thing—kept me motivated. I just had to find a way to spread my message.

With both sentences, what's next?

It didn't take me long to figure it out.

Social media.

* * *

Into the night—at home and in my bedroom—I built the Facebook profile. I used the name of Jessica Wilmer, loosely based on Jesus and Will. I made the profile's intro "no one," and excluded personal information.

I have to be unattached to the words—they alone must create the shift in people's minds.

As I worked, something unexplainable happened. My smartphone screen flashed. Random apps bounced around like a pinball machine. Loading times increased significantly.

Are computer gods trying to stop me again?

It made sense. I never feared an accident of my own accord or a natural disaster. But mechanically composed electrical currents were something different.

After hours of battling with beings hiding in the wavelengths, the profile was set up.

Now, to share the truth.

To sum up my purpose with social media, I posted an image stating, "The mind of one freethinker can possess a million ideas. A million fanatics can have their minds possessed by a single idea."

I then wondered how to share the sentences.

On the floor, I found a piece of paper with black and white lines stuck in a square. It resembled society as a chaotic swirl of paths that could never be set free. Therefore, the world was limited in what it could achieve. With the truth, however, the box could open and guide the paths to the best possible destination.

What is the best possible destination, though?

I thought in the context of positive direction on a line graph. Society has typically viewed the idea of progress in the right and upward direction. If "human needs" was the *x*-axis and "prosperity" was the *y*-axis, then the more "human needs" being met, the more "prosperity."

This has rung true as we have sought more—whether material wealth or power-driven abilities such as technology and medicine. However, we have had more than we would ever need, right?

Where do we go then?

A lightbulb clicked. To find the best possible destination for everyone, we must rethink prosperity. We must look at what we have and determine how to grow with each other.

One could see that, if we have more than we need, more "human needs" would not mean more "prosperity." But if needs were met by more people, we'd all have more prosperity.

We'd all have more prosperity.

Instead of right and upward on the graph, we must look left and upward.

But how to inspire that shift?

A test. As the universe did for me, I would give clues on the profile. If others solved it, they would discover the answers.

I wrote the eternal life sentence on one paper and the fraternity sentence on another (shown on page 197). Eternal life—on the right—would always exist, while fraternity—on the left—had to be achieved. I angled the fraternity paper inward because it needed action.

I tested the conjunction between "thinking" and "doing" for the fraternity sentence by adding three question marks with the optional answers of "and," "or," and "then." To have fraternity, one would have to think before doing. Therefore, once they chose "then," the correct conjunction, one form of the truth would be known.

For the other truth, another step was required.

How can fraternity become eternal?

When turning the fraternity paper to the left, the sentences would align. This would show how we have shifted our view of progress the other way. For this step's clue, I posted a video scanning from the right to the left, setting up my shot to include a transition from darkness to light.

Now...to connect with others.

I friend-requested as many people as possible. Soon enough, I connected to dozens of others, and the feed was filled with arbitrary images and messages.

Another avenue for signs from the universe.

Around three in the morning, I scrolled upon an illustration of a couple being affectionate (Figure 4). One after the other, similar images presented themselves.

It was time.

She's waiting for me at the church.

Inescapable illusion.

* * *

I had been questioning life's meaning since I became unwell. I was hopeless when running ended—insecure when Humanities stimulated existential dread. I pursued my theory to heal—philosophy inspired me. But it was driven by illness.

Psychosis is often described as a condition where someone loses contact with reality. But losing contact with reality would mean we know what reality truly is.

My psychosis was my reality. Everything I was doing, thinking, and feeling was real. Therefore, I see reality as more abstruse—perhaps something reliant on the perception and/or experience of each thing. However, my reality was likely to disrupt the orderly state of humankind.

I believe challenging society's standards, such as what prosperity means, can help us grow. But being bound to a reality so distorted is not healthy.

What if a sign led me to something terrible?

Now, I know I was delusional the entire time. My ex-girlfriend was never going to marry me. I wasn't shifting people's views by connecting with them. I wasn't changing the world with my theory.

What was my theory anyway? Was I onto something, or was I just exploring philosophical thought? Either way, shouldn't my health and wellness have come first?

More than half of those with schizophrenia believe they are God, the devil, a prophet, or another important person. But everyone's experience is different.

In the end, psychosis trapped me—that was it. I couldn't control my thoughts or behavior without understanding the symptoms. As I journeyed further into the delusional story, help was more unlikely.

Would I get a second chance?

DERAILED CHAOS

I ran out of the house in the dead air of three in the morning. My noisy steps woke up my dad.

"What are you doing?" he asked, following me to my car.

"I have to go to the church with the big red doors," I said.

He looked confused and worried. But I moved quickly. He couldn't stop me from igniting the car and speeding off.

It felt like Judgment Day was on the horizon. The sky was pitch black. My car lights scorched the shadows of the road.

Racing one hundred miles per hour, I had to get to the church as soon as possible.

She's waiting for me.

"You have to go faster. Faster," static-like voices from the radio said. "You're gonna miss your chance!"

But I remained confident.

Everyone in the world is waiting for this. It's going to happen.

I pictured the moment I'd burst into the hall—white light and familiar faces. My wife would jump in my arms and secure our marriage with a kiss. It'd be the resolution scene—a happily ever after.

When I arrived, cop cars lined the street. A few men in black stood on the sidewalk.

Must be a test.

I could outrun them.

Screech. My car squealed as I stopped and sprinted to the big red doors.

The cops chased me. But I was in the main hall by the time they reached the steps. I was standing in dark emptiness, stupefied.

How can this be? Where is she?

Seconds later, blistering light seared my eyes—suspended white circles billowing in the black. Loud voices subdued my next move.

"What are you doing here?" a man in black shouted.

They grabbed my arm and shuffled me to the door. Once I saw my car in the distance, I broke their grip. But this time, I wasn't fast enough.

They snagged my body, pulling my limbs toward the ground.

"I am God!" I shouted, standing tall until I fell weak—my face smashing into the dirt.

The next thing I knew, I was in the back of a cop car—silver cuffs tightened my wrists.

Another test.

I threw my elbow at the window. I scrambled on the floor for a key.

But nope—no way out.

What went wrong?

* * *

A cop drove us off—town lights disappearing as the ominous country roads rumbled under my feet. I looked for my next clue, leaning towards the partition. The lucent dashboard drew me in—buttons and knobs I'd never seen before.

Is he really a cop?

"I was pretty fast, wasn't I?" I said. "I used to run and do triathlons."

"I've done triathlons, too," he said. "Someday, I want to do an Ironman."

An Ironman—like Coach Dan.

My eyes lit up.

I must be on the right path.

All of a sudden, I was in a room with white walls, white floors, and scattered hints of yellow and blue. Free from handcuffs, I explored the chilly, bright area that looked like a waiting room—rocklike couches and a TV hoisted in the corner. A transparent barrier covered the ledge of a tall, long desk.

Have I been here before?

I glued my face to the desk's blockade to inspect the details behind it.

"Folders," a little blue label said. F O L D E R S.

I fold...what? Hers? Furs?

"Oh, so you're just going to stare at that," a man in blue said from the other side.

I didn't know what to say. I walked away.

Does he not know who I am?

I wandered into a space where others in street clothes stood around. An elderly man, looking distraught, sat on a couch. His raggedy shirt, patches of long white hair, and missing teeth reminded me of the first man I saw without a home.

I was a child on a trip to Toronto with my dad. While getting on a bus, a man stood near—his eyes depleted and desperate. His appearance—dirty and wearing tattered clothes, the plea for help apparent on his sign—sunk my young heart.

I couldn't help the man near the bus, but maybe, I could help the man on the couch. So, I sat near him—his musty shirt reminiscent of my visits to Grandma.

"Why are you here?" I asked.

"I've been ill for a long time," he said. "I don't know if I can continue to live."

I was sad.

No one should feel despair in this world.

I held his hands, kept my posture toward him, and continued to listen. He talked about his addiction, homelessness, and so on. When the moment was right, I used my theory to respond.

"Your feelings come from your thoughts and what you are doing," I said. "What you are doing is sitting here with me. Your thoughts, well, you can change them right now. No matter where you've come from or what you've done, think about what you are doing here—being with me."

The elderly man's face lit up with a radiant smile.

"You saved me," he said as tears fell. "Thank you, sir, thank you."

I couldn't help but smile too.

Did I heal him with my touch and voice? Am I like Jesus?

"Yes, yes, yes…you're a healer," voices from the TV said. "You're meant to heal people."

A new ability.

* * *

I didn't know when I last slept. After exerting so much energy helping the elderly man, my exhaustion took charge.

"Is there a place I can sleep?" I asked a woman behind the desk.

"You have to wait. It'll be a while," she said.

Why do I have to wait? Does she not know who I am?

"The prophet, although trapped by the fears of society, has shown his greatest gift," I heard the TV say. "When will they all believe?"

My anxiety increased as every minute passed. After what felt like an eternity, the woman at the desk called me back.

"Take this," she said, sliding a small cup with a tiny white pill through a gap in the barrier.

"What is it?" I asked.

"It'll help you sleep."

That's all I want.

I swallowed the pill. Soon after, a different woman stepped out from the desk, telling me to follow her. She had voluptuous curves and brown hair draping down her backside.

When she turned to me and pointed to a bedroom, I paused.

"Don't I know you?" I asked.

"No, you don't," she said.

"You were in the hospital a few weeks back, right?"

"Nope," she said, avoiding eye contact. "I've always been here."

Oh…I get it.

She couldn't reveal herself. She was an observer—someone who did believe in me.

I held the secret in as I entered the bedroom. Everything was white as expected—nothing worthy to note. However, when lying down, the window caught my attention.

Sharp lines of moonlight formed a symmetrical pattern from the outdoors to my bed. Although the moon's perfectly round and luminous existence floated in the distance, I felt close enough to touch it.

I am on the right path.

Would this time be different?

* * *

I awoke to find myself on a couch in the main room. My dad and mom sat nearby, talking with each other. When they saw I was awake, their heads turned, and their eyes widened.

It felt like they knew exactly what was happening. But I had no idea how I ended up on that couch.

I closed my eyes, wanting to sleep more.

"You need to stay awake," my dad said.

"Why?"

"Because the doctor is coming to see you," my mom added.

I rolled my eyes, dragging my body up, so I didn't doze off. In a white coat, the doctor appeared and pulled us into a separate room. Disoriented and slow, my staggered steps followed.

The space felt awkward.

What are we doing here?

I zoned out while the man talked with my parents. But he then looked at me.

"What do you see?" he asked—his thick accent hanging low in the insipid room.

"Color coordination," I said, trying to shake off the cobwebs of deep sleep.

He looked content and pulled out an orange container with pills in it.

"Take one each night, he said. "You can cut the tablet in half if you want to."

I nodded in agreement—my muffled mind couldn't care less at that point.

As we left the room, I expected to stay—perhaps go back to bed. But when my parents said I was going with them, a hopeful force sprung me back to life.

Onto the next step.

* * *

I couldn't recall any part of the building. When I stepped into the fresh air, blue arrows painted on a cement wall nearby pointed in the same direction. I assumed we'd follow them.

When my dad drove out of the parking garage in his blue car, I was correct.

The signs are correct.

For the entire drive home, I silently stared at the sunset. Its sharp, distinct circle with a goldish round edge reminded me of the rings I'd put on my wife and me.

Sunday had to be the day of our wedding. The fact it was God's day made perfect sense.

How did I not realize that before?

With the wedding two days away, I wanted to spend quality time with my parents. Once I left to travel the world and share my word, I didn't know how much I'd see them.

I'll miss them.

I planned to watch a movie with my dad, particularly the SpongeBob SquarePants movie. As a child, he helped me decorate my bedroom with SpongeBob merch—curtains, blankets, and linen sewn on a bean bag chair. He enjoyed the show as much as I did.

I placed my phone on the ottoman at the room's center and angled its camera toward me—the ideal location for everyone to witness what was happening. Based on my Facebook profile, the world could see and hear me through my smartphone.

Keeping in mind the professor's study of me—the prophet—I welcomed their observations.

As the movie began, I felt nostalgia like never before. SpongeBob's energy and positivity were inspiring. Every animation and voiceover was directed to me—as if the movie was made for me that night.

In the scene when SpongeBob was leaving his home for the journey ahead, I heard my dad crying. I knew he'd miss me. I was sure to say *I love you* before bed that night.

But I have to go, Dad.

I wasn't alone. The movie's plot and my own were the same.

SpongeBob had to embark on a mission to retrieve King Neptune's crown. In hopes of stealing the secret formula, Plankton—the evil plankton—sent the crown to Shell City, so he could enslave Bikini Bottom.

Everyone doubted SpongeBob, saying he was just a kid. But his optimism overcame. He completed the mission and rescued everyone.

My hope thrived. No matter how arduous my mission was, humanity would be victorious.

Just like SpongeBob getting the crown and saving the town.

* * *

I visited my mom the next day. She was babysitting my four-year-old nephew. Anytime we were together, he wanted to play.

We made forts. We raced toy cars and created a mini restaurant, making pizza and tacos for stuffed animals. Something was so beautiful about the simple joy he had with the world. I felt I was there, engaging in a childhood I left so long ago.

When I sat with my mom, life felt old. She talked about work, stress...the weather.

A credit card commercial snagged my attention. Looking sleek and modern, it presented traditional ideals of wealth and power—suits, shiny jewelry, and high-tech equipment. The recognizable actor and his profound voice spoke to me and my mission.

"Now tell me, what's in your wallet," he said, talking about the Quicksilver card.

I need that card.

"Shouldn't the Ten Commandments read 'Thou shalt not want or have to steal…Thou shalt not want or have to kill,' and so forth?" I asked my mom. "Isn't it about creating a world where sins are less likely to weigh on one's mind than being told not to commit?"

"Uh…I'm not sure, Cohen," she said.

I was unsure where the sudden revelation came from. But I took a mental note. Every bit of knowledge was going to help me succeed in my mission.

"What were you saying about work, Mom?"

* * *

I returned to my dad's to rest before the wedding. Later in the night, an ad for gold rings appeared on my Facebook.

How could I forget?

I asked my dad if he had any, telling him I wanted to propose to Carrie.

"Didn't you break up?" he asked.

"We're getting back together."

Initially, he may have been confused, but extending the family was important.

"That's great news," he smiled, "Grandma might have a ring."

Grandma's house was a quick drive. When I arrived and told her about my proposal, she smiled too.

"Oh, that's so nice, Cohen. I can't wait to meet her," she said. "There might be some upstairs. A wooden box with a flower on it."

I frantically searched, feeling like I was in a maze. For as long as I knew my grandma, she hoarded items—furniture and clutter strewed about. When I found the box, inside were discolored rings and a sparkling blue earring.

I questioned if I had interpreted the sign correctly—they were supposed to be gorgeous gold rings.

Maybe someone else would bring them to the wedding?

I grabbed the blue earring instead and returned home.

"Did she have any?" my dad asked.

"No, but that's okay," I said. "I don't need them right now."

To avoid any more confusion, I sought comfort in my bedroom. As I readied for bed, a sign cleared everything up.

"Goodnight, Dad."

"Goodnight," he said, sniffling.

At that moment, the TV revealed a person kneeling before a gravestone.

"Just touch it," a voice whispered.

Just touch the grave?

The second of these thoughts, my Facebook showed videos and pictures of brotherly love. A man lifted himself out of the ground and hugged another. A face resembled my dad's longing to be reunited.

My uncle.

The grave of my dad's brother was on a hill nearby.

I could bring him back to life, so my dad would be happy.

Resurrecting trauma.

* * *

Throughout the night, I prepared for the wedding. I put on the blue earring. I dressed in my all-black suit. I found a red Christmas tie I stole for a holiday-themed party in college. Its snowflakes signified forgiveness and my ability to overcome.

I was ready to go by 1:00 a.m. The second I resorted to my Facebook, an illustration appeared.

"I hear wedding bells," the image said, displaying a picture of two gold bells with a blue ribbon tying them together.

Time to go.

I didn't want to wake up my dad. Therefore, I snuck out my bedroom window, quietly lifting its pane and stepping outside.

Wait…the Quicksilver card.

I recalled how my dad kept one in his wallet. I used my phone's flashlight to search for it in the kitchen until I remembered he sometimes kept his wallet in his car.

Test intensifies.

I went back out the window—the deep silence warm and soft. In my dad's car, I found the wallet and card.

I knew it. Test complete.

I quietly started my car in the still night and slowly pulled out of the driveway. My car creaked and crackled—its axles bending with the wheels turning. On the road, I tapped the brakes to stop. I wanted to look at my home one last time.

My dad was a skilled handyman. Attached to the roof, he built a wooden pergola that overhung our front windows. Underneath it was a path of white pebbles edged off from the front lawn.

I remembered my dad teaching me to cut grass. My little body—half his height—scanned the mower's engine, trying to find the red gasoline button.

"Pump that three times," he'd say, before letting me rip the pull cord.

I'm going to miss living here.

I didn't want to leave my dad, it was sad. But I had to.

Change had to come.

I'll love you forever, Dad. See you soon.

* * *

The dark and secluded sky comforted me as I drove. I fantasized about the wedding—lines of every vibrant color gleaning from the church's stained windows. Inside, glistening lights would mimic daytime.

"All things bright and beautiful...Love is divine, all love excels...," I heard choir music sing through my car's radio.

Everyone is waiting for me.

Less than a hundred feet before the church, I passed a tattoo parlor with a single light on.

My sentences.

I walked to the parlor—the street was deserted except for distant cheering from the church.

They'll have to wait.

Stepping to a door, I heard voices from the other side and knocked.

"Hey, man, what's up?" a man my age answered.

"I need a tattoo," I said.

"Sure, man, come on in," he said with a slight chuckle.

Beer cans and bongs filled the room. Weed smoke engulfed the air. A man, who was supposedly the tattoo artist, sat nearby.

"I need a tattoo right now."

I described my sentences aligned down the center of my spine.

"You're fucking high, dude," the artist said.

No, I'm not.

Pulling out the Quicksilver card, I said, "What about this?"

"No, dude. I don't want your money."

I kept pressing. He kept saying no. At one point, he raised a fist in my face.

"Get the fuck out of here, man!"

I didn't understand.

Why couldn't the tattoo be done? I followed the signs.

I listened, however. I didn't want any conflict, and time was moving fast.

Tick, tick, tick…I have to get to the church.

As I left, I learned the real reason why I had to go to the parlor. The interruption of my journey allowed me to see how messy my car was.

This isn't worthy of my wife.

I rapidly cleaned it, throwing away weeks' worth of trash—fast food scraps, crinkled-up wrapping papers, and baggies. I found my notebook and class textbooks.

I don't need these anymore. I know everything.

I tossed them into the street bin. I then stumbled upon my passport.

The world knows who I am, right?

I ripped out my license and tore it into pieces. I threw away everything in my wallet, tearing up anything with my name, except the Quicksilver card.

People knew me by my words—not my name.

No longer am I tied to what society has made of me.

No longer was I me.

* * *

I was in crisis for days. I was fortunate to go to the hospital—again. But one night was far from enough to provide me with the support I needed.

Again, I'm not surprised how I responded to treatment and the results. The system can work in getting people to a place for support but oftentimes struggles to actually provide support. A tiresome frustration I feel every day, continuing to see how much the system fails so many who need help.

During my stay, a nurse practitioner, social worker, and psychiatrist evaluated me. Their notes described my first hospital visit and potential diagnoses. I talked about seeing signs and how the world watched me. But they still had reason to let me go.

> *This is a young man who exhibits mild delusional beliefs but did not exhibit any concerning symptoms that would warrant continued observation. Patient was offered voluntary admission but declined and agreed to start meds.*

Apparently, I denied symptoms of hallucinations and severe mania. I told the doctors I enjoyed college and would graduate soon. It's like I was still there, functioning as my typical self, yet a distorted reality mastered my consciousness.

My parents denied safety concerns. Exhaustion due to days of not sleeping quieted me. It felt easier to say I was okay than to explain my truth.

Again, no one's at fault. I don't blame the treatment providers or my parents. It was easy for me to fall through the cracks. The issues are systemic and go beyond any individual.

How can you deny someone's feelings about themselves? With physical illness, people are more likely to tell you they're not okay. For mental illness, it's the opposite.

I don't recall declining to stay, but why would I have wanted to stay? I rejected my illness and treatment. I had no understanding of mental health and wasn't capable of talking about my symptoms.

My family continued misinterpreting my behavior. Watching a movie and playing with my nephew were signs of healthy functioning.

When I asked for the rings, why weren't my father or grandmother concerned? They knew I dated Carrie for a long time, and it's typical to be excited about marriage. So was this request so unusual that they should have been concerned?

Some warning signs, like driving one hundred miles per hour and almost fighting a tattoo artist, could not be seen by family or treatment providers. However, the treatment providers knew I had delusional beliefs and an early history of mental illness. They knew at 3:00 a.m., the police picked me up at a church.

What could've been different for me to stay in the hospital?

My mental illness was just noticed—would it have been reasonable to keep me out of caution and further explore my insight? What about the hospital environment was ineffective? How do you justify violating my right to deny treatment—should the Mental Hygiene Law include a more intensive evaluation for psychosis-related illness?

Voluntary versus involuntary admission into the hospital is complex. Regardless, doctors released me with severe symptoms.

We missed our second chance.

INFERNAL DECEPTION

I walked the pathway to the church. When I arrived at its doors, I paused. The red paint's glossy texture smoldered against the night's shadow.

Why is it so quiet?

I held my breath. I squeezed the handle—the bronze dampening my fingers with midnight dew. I pushed.

The doors did not budge.

How are they locked?

Every time I was there, they opened at my will.

Perhaps I have something left to do.

Around the church, I found an unlocked door lit by a single light. I stepped into a room resembling a smaller, more vibrant version of the main hall.

Gentle, yellow light coated the shiny railings and precise woodwork of the pews. In the front, chalices of silver and gold sat on an intricate white cloth. A plush red carpet with an extravagant pattern covered the floor.

I took off my shoes and sat in the front pew. I relaxed my hands and feet—the heated air comforting my bones. With deep breathing, I let my worries go, feeling more at peace with every minute.

Chirp…chirp…chirp. A bird consistently whistled from outside a window.

After an hour or so, it felt like the bird was waiting for me to do something. I then saw a sheet of paper next to me. I cautiously grabbed it, hoping I was doing the right thing. On it were ten or so statements.

I must prepare for when they come.

"For God so loved the world that he gave his one and only Son, that whoever believes in him shall not perish but have eternal life." I read. "For God did not send his Son into the world to condemn the world, but in order that the world might be saved through him."

Over and over, I repeated the verses until I memorized them. Once confident, I knelt on the carpet in the center of the room.

"God, give me the strength to carry out my mission," I whispered.

I felt strong and calm—a purity interconnecting my being with the universe. It didn't take me long to realize what I had to do.

I must join the sufferings of Jesus Christ.

I pulled my arms and legs behind my back, forcing my head toward the floor. My body cracked and bent. My feet and hands shook. It felt like I had grown in size—amazed at my ability to morph into impossible forms.

I could never achieve this before.

After many minutes, I released my arms and legs. Everything but my head went numb. A sensation lifted me off the ground.

My body is sacrificed, rising into the eternal.

My mind was next. I crossed my legs underneath me. I closed my eyes. I took the nail of my pointer finger and gouged my forehead's center. I felt it cut through my skin and into my skull, blood trickling down my face.

As the nail reached my brain, the bird's chirp fainted. I was drifting into the underworld. When the chirp vanished, I put my hands together at my chest.

The sacrifice is complete.

Life was empty yet full. I was suspended in a place where all things were and all things were not.

I'm in the unknown.

*Creeeak...*A door softly opened.

Delicate, mysterious steps shuffled around me. The moment they went silent, I brought my spirit onto the pew. More steps arrived as the spirits of the underworld surrounded me. Without sight, I felt their presence.

"He is here. He is here," they whispered. "Praise him, for he has succeeded."

A man addressed us—his deep voice filled the room.

"We are here today, for the Son has returned. Join me as we restore the body and blood of our Lord, God, and Savior Jesus Christ."

I'm gonna be reincarnated.

He continued to speak words of prophecy and the rebirth of the chosen one. Energized senses pulsed within me.

Matter. Chatter. Scatter.

It's working.

"And this is eternal life," the others sang in harmony. "That they may know You, the only true God..."

I vibrated with ecstasy—life flashing through my veins. The ensemble ascended my soul. Once it found my body, I felt my bones begin to mend and my forehead seal.

I'm returning.

The man directed the congregation to the last step.

"Time to consume the body and blood of Jesus."

Of me.

Eyes still closed, I sensed the man collect the blood from my face and scoop marrow from my still-soft bone. The others lined up. One by one, they consumed what I provided.

I felt a split-second where I could see into the underworld, opening my eyes to glance behind my shoulder. My late grandfather was looking at me—teary eyes shining with love. I hadn't seen him since I was three. My dad sat behind him.

They're both here for me—a bloodline of humble divinity supporting the return of Jesus.

I closed my eyes as the man said his final words.

"Mass has ended. Go in peace to love and serve the Lord."

Everyone stood up. I felt enough life to return to my usual state and opened my eyes.

My being is certain.

My brain was bleeding.

* * *

My dad walked to me. I had been at the church for many hours.

"How did you know I was here?" I asked.

"You mentioned wanting to go, and I wanted to come too," he said. "Your car was gone when I woke up, so I figured you were here."

Perfect timing.

I didn't have much more to say. I felt worn out and tired. When we neared the back exit of the church, he handed me his smartphone, saying I should talk with my mom.

"Are you okay, Cohen?" she asked. "Why did you go to church?"

"Yes, I am okay," I said. "I just wanted to go to church."

The morning air embraced me like I was born again. Several times my dad asked me if I was going straight home.

"Yes, Dad, I am fine," I repeated. "I will be home soon"

After he left, I leaned back in my car's snug seat. I pulled out the blue earring, feeling some relief.

Everything had a reason. But what is next?

...

Duh!

I still had to get married.

How did I forget?

My mind was fully activated as I ran into the church. Since I entered through the back door this time, I had to find my way to the main hall.

Another maze.

I followed a series of hallways, echoes of choir music guiding me. I discovered a room with gold and silver chalices, candle sticks, and bells.

Are the gold rings here?

I couldn't find them. But a cross earring caught my eye. Green, yellow, blue, and red gems were placed at its ends—a symbol that my life was in harmonious balance.

I found a space with tall brown doors. Slightly opening them, I saw a choir singing and a single face smiling at me.

The wedding is finally happening!

I swung open the doors, standing still in the main hall's front area. Dozens of people lined up in the pews facing me. Women in dresses. Men in buttoned-up shirts.

I had one problem though. No one looked familiar.

A man in the front row waved for me to sit beside him. I followed.

"That must have been pretty embarrassing," he said.

I didn't respond—I had no reason to be embarrassed.

Unless I have dried blood on my face from the sacrifice.

I never cleaned the healed puncture. Plus, I was wearing a black suit with a red tie.

Do I look evil?

Everyone suddenly stood up. The man handed me an open Bible, and people began singing. He moved his finger with the verses, encouraging me to join.

But where is my wife-to-be?

She never showed. The priest then directed everyone to consume the body and blood of Jesus.

Am I about to consume myself?

The man escorted me through kneeling, crossing my face and chest, and consuming. After eating the body and blood, I realized I wasn't consuming myself but the self in a state of pure sanctity. Although I knew about the sacrifice, no one else did. Therefore, I had to consume to represent that self.

I had to be what I was to show others what they could be.

* * *

The service ended. With no sign of what to do next, I left the church.

I drove home, pondering what I had missed. I was wrong about the wedding. I was wrong about traveling the world to spread the truth. I was alone.

I spent the evening looking for signs. But with none, I sought sleep. However, a pain in my head throbbed, and I couldn't shut my thoughts off. It felt like something was preventing me from resting.

I tried techniques to help. I counted numbers and letters. I pictured water dripping into a puddle. I made my body symmetrical and put my hands in prayer, feeling my chest rise and drop.

Soon enough, I nodded off. In what felt like a minute later, I shot out of bed. It was morning, and my dad was gone.

With inspiring energy, I turned on the TV and saw naked people dancing. Their pale skin was smooth, and their thin bodies moved like arches floating in the sky.

Gods.

I undressed and went into the bathroom. While examining my body, I saw a bubble on my toe. Underneath it, gold blood sparkled.

I am a God. My first step since being reborn was to sleep.

I readied the shower, thinking of shaving off my hair. But then, I saw a paper ball in the toilet—blood seeping from its cracks.

Cancer was in my family's genes.

How did I not know about my dad's cancer?

Sweat dripped down my brow.

Did I lose sight of my family?

Crash! I jumped two feet as a horrifying sound rang from the shower.

I looked in to see a small mirror on the floor—its black back toward me. I flipped it and three cracks in the glass split my face into thirds.

What has happened to me?

* * *

Gray clouds hovered in the sky. I drove to the church, wondering again if today would be the big day. Instead of a suit, I wore a green shirt with a four-leaf clover design.

I need some luck.

I made it to the big red doors and peered my head in. As expected, the hall was empty. Remaining hopeful, I went to the smaller room where my self-sacrifice occurred. But again, no one was around.

Why is this so hard?

I did the only thing I could think of and prayed.

"I'm sorry I never touched my uncle's grave. I'm sorry I have focused too much on myself and not my family."

I pulled the cross earring from my pocket and placed it on the altar.

"I am sorry I stole from the church," I added.

I began to walk out when I realized I never wore the earring.

Maybe that's what went wrong?

I grabbed it before leaving. I then drove to the only place I could think of—home. On my way, my mom called. But her voice was broken up by cracking sound waves.

"Go…there…Cohen…," I heard.

I hung up the second I knew what she meant. I drove to a restaurant called Steve's Place. Steven was my middle name, and the building was white with red trim—a novel look. The sign's design included a silver knife.

The devil must live underneath. He's trying to disguise himself.

But I knew better. To show the devil I could get rid of him, I smashed a building's window and tossed in red items including a hat, lighter, and an Old Spice container. I whacked my car's tail lights with an ice scraper, pinching my fingers underneath to pull apart broken pieces.

What's next?

I pierced my ear with the cross earring. Dark red blood dripped on my shirt. I feared harming the green, so I sucked on the spot. But that only doubled my panic.

Gods are not supposed to bleed. And I just consumed red!

Feeling terrified, I paced back and forth in the parking lot.

"What did I just do?" I shouted. "What do I do?"

I spotted a large blue bin with a white symbol in the back of Steve's Place.

Maybe my sentences go in there.

As I had done on Facebook, I wrote the puzzle of my sentences on a paper slip. I stuffed it in a yellow sock—one from my first hospital visit—and dropped it in the bin.

I'm not strong enough. Someone else must finish the mission.

I continued home. Since removing all of the taillights took too long, I ditched my car at a junkyard. The second I parked in the field of beat-up vehicles, I threw my keys into the wide open—I didn't want to find them. I then searched for a car with no red when, suddenly, my dad called.

"Why didn't you go to work?" he demanded. "Where are you?"

"I…uh…" I stuttered. "I'm at that junkyard outside of town."

He urged me to get home, saying he'd meet me there. However, I couldn't drive because I couldn't find my keys.

"Call Grandma, and she'll pick you up," he said.

I listened.

* * *

My grandma and I waited for my dad at home. I wandered around, struggling to breathe. I didn't know what to do—my thoughts felt jumbled and murky.

When my dad arrived, his bright red face contrasted with his black work uniform. He was flailing his hands—dark eyes filled with anger.

"What are you doing? Why didn't you go to school or work?"

The fury in his voice made me uncomfortable. I tried answering his questions, but I struggled to speak words.

Does he not know about the wedding or my mission?

"You need to go back to the fucking hospital," he said as he picked up the phone.

I felt afraid, so I searched for a sign. I scanned my surroundings. I looked at Facebook.

My heart beat faster and faster with each second. Like the end of a major race, it felt like I was upon a defining moment that would determine my fate.

What is next?

My dad handed me the phone.

"What's going on? Are you okay? Why didn't you go to work?" my mom asked.

"I…uh…"

An unfamiliar voice emerged on the line.

"What's going on? Are you okay?" a woman claiming to be a police officer asked.

The same fucking questions over and over again—I wanted to scream. Everyone seemed worried, frustrated, and annoyed. But no one was helping.

What am I supposed to do?

I retreated to the living room to gather my thoughts. Not long after, a series of signs gave me an answer.

A message appeared on Facebook Messenger. It read, "Satan: hahahaha…" followed by a conversation in French (shown on page 197).

You don't fool me, Satan. I'll show you.

I then received a friend request. Their profile picture illustrated a person smashing their hands on another person—an angry ghost flying out of their head. Dots of yellow and orange were at the collision point (shown on page 198).

I get it.

The puzzle pieces fit together. His black clothes. His red face. His cancer.

The devil is inside my dad.

It all made sense. But could I face the unimaginable—the unconscionable? Could I succeed in the ultimate test of God? Could I kill my dad to rid the devil of this world?

"This can't be the next step. This can't be the next step!" I shouted, pacing around the living room. "There has to be another way. I can't do this."

But the sign is clear. The devil is inside my dad, and he will die anyway.

* * *

I walked into the kitchen where my dad and grandma remained. I opened a drawer. Right on top was a silver knife with a white handle—the holiest of colors. I grabbed it and slowly stepped near my dad, pondering how to make the move.

"What are you doing, Cohen?" he asked, slightly backing away.

But my eyes were black, and I was detached, feeling like a raging animal with one goal.

Complete the mission.

I lunged at him. The knife soared through the air, gunning for his chest. He responded fast, knocking it out of my hand.

We began shoving each other. Time picked up the pace as our movements were quick and sudden, muscle against muscle; my dad wasn't weak.

We tumbled to the ground, and he pinned me on the floor. I couldn't move my arms, so I clamped my jaw on the lower part of his ear. My teeth sunk through—blood dripped, staining our shirts.

"Ahhh!" he shrieked, getting off of me and walking away.

"I have to do this," I grumbled, pausing to rest.

When I obtained the strength to stand, I looked for the knife. However, my grandma had put it back in the drawer. So, I searched the house for something else.

My dad had been remodeling.

I found a red screwdriver, a black hammer, and a yellow wrench. But nothing white.

I have to use that knife.

I returned to the kitchen to see my dad hunched over the counter—arms straight, head down, heavy panting. My grandma was near the knife drawer—stunned in shock.

The second they saw me, I made my move.

"Block the drawer!" my dad screamed.

But she was too late. I snagged the knife and ran at my dad again.

"Don't kill your father," she wept. "Don't kill your father!"

Do I have to kill her too?!

Thankfully, she wore a green shirt.

I lunged at my dad, hoping to finally complete the mission. But he seized my arms and shoved me against the wall. I shimmied my hands underneath his shoulders—enough space to thrust the knife toward his throat.

The second the blade tip neared his neck, he wedged his thumb in between. No matter how hard I pushed, it wouldn't puncture.

I lost strength and leaned back, breathing deeply. Remaining deadlocked, time paused. I looked down to see my dad's bushy white hair. Its tender bristles brushed against my face.

What the fuck am I doing?

All of a sudden, he disappeared.

I froze.

Where did he go?

Once the thought of him dead hit me, my throat choked up, and my stomach dropped.

"What did I do," I yelled.

What did I do?

I ran through the house.

"I'm sorry, Dad, I'm sorry!" I shrieked.

Guilt and shame gushed through me like wildfire. I couldn't find him.

I looked at Facebook for an answer. A picture of a grave appeared.

Oh my God…he's gone.

He was gone.

"I'm sorry, Dad," I screamed as I ran outside. "Forgive me, I'm sorry!"

"Get down now," someone shouted. "Get down now, or we will shoot!"

I turned around. Two men in black pointed guns at me.

I raised my hands, still holding my phone.

"Drop that and get on the ground!" they shouted.

I listened.

Moments later, I was in the backseat of a car—silver rings binding my wrists and ankles. When those in black stopped questioning me, I looked toward my home.

My dad stood on the front steps—blood drops dotted his shirt.

He's alive. Thank you, God. He's alive.

A miracle.

* * *

Imagine where I would be now if that knife punctured my father's throat. He wouldn't be here. I'd be locked up somewhere. Psychosis still tormenting me.

I had no intention of hurting him. But what pisses me off the most is that I was unwell for more than a year. I was in and out of the hospital throughout the month. I was in crisis for a week—days of pure chaos before I tried to kill him.

How was this not preventable?

Again, anything could have happened. Instead, I became the next poster child for violence and mental illness. I'd be criminalized and feared rather than given empathy and support—just like many others with mental illness.

I can't express how fortunate I am that we survived. My father survived. Even my grandma escaped death by the color of her shirt.

When my father told me the cops almost shot me because they thought I held a gun, not a phone, I was paralyzed with horror. If social conditioning hadn't allowed my sanity to return at that moment, I might've been killed.

I wouldn't be here. I wouldn't be writing these words. I'd probably be seen as another fucking crazy person whose life is unworthy of being with everyone else.

But I am here. I am healthy. Now, I feel bitter at the display of heartlessness. Violence due to untreated mental illness is just a tragic result of our society's failure to adequately support mental health.

When asked about my behavior leading up to the incident, my father said, "I was worried. But you said you were fine. The doctors said you were on pot, but they agreed you were fine too.

That made me feel okay even if I was still worried. Now, I don't know how they agreed. They should've known."

We shouldn't have had to rely on a miracle to survive, but it was far too late to prevent what happened. The cops took me to jail where the severity of my illness increased. The guilt I felt from attacking my father and my relief of his life being saved wasn't enough to quiet my psychosis.

What would my symptoms do next?

THE DARK ABYSS

A man in black drove me away from my house. I squished my body against the car window, seeking comfort in the fields of trees, grass, and rolling hills. Color dissipated as shadowy clouds dulled the land.

I didn't know where I was going, and it didn't matter. Life felt over.

When the car parked, the man opened the back door and grabbed my shoulder. He pulled me into a building and cuffed my ankles to a white steel bench.

Sweat hovered in the large, bitter-looking office. The stale air smelled greasy. A dozen people in matching black shuffled around.

I didn't recognize anyone or feel welcome. Even when the people weren't staring at me with outrage, they looked stressed.

Chattering. Electrical noises. Computers dinging and phones ringing.

How could anyone be happy here?

I wanted to leave. I wanted silence. I wanted to see my dad.

Voices from a TV in the corner captured my angst.

"How could he do that to his father?" the news anchors said. "We were lied to. He wasn't the one."

I felt sick.

"Can we turn the TV off?" I asked the man at a desk near me.

"Yeah…okay, sir," he said, chuckling as he rolled his eyes.

It was official. My mission failed. I couldn't come back.

What is next? Death?

* * *

I fantasized about death. However, it would have to be final this time. I didn't want to be revived in the same body.

When we were young, Finn and I would hike up a large hill near Cohocton. We'd dip our heads under a small row of trees, stepping to a stone cliff to peer over. Several hundred feet of sunless space separated its ledge and the bottom of the abyss.

A beautiful place to die.

I wanted to fall through the black, bitter air of my night to come. I wouldn't know where I was going, and it didn't matter.

"I have to sacrifice myself," I said to the man at the desk.

"We wouldn't want you to do that," he replied, not making eye contact.

But I wanted to. I felt at peace. My memories of the places I had been and the people I had met—I was okay with it all being gone.

I can't live after what I did to my dad.

"Where is my dad?" I asked.

"He's in the hospital. You did a number on him," he said. "You should be ashamed."

* * *

A man in black unfastened me from the bench and directed me to the corner of the room. Others took my picture and pasted my fingerprints onto a computer screen. They had to try multiple times. Technology struggled to capture my presence.

Am I evil now?

A man in black led me to a small, dreary room with no windows. Two men sat across from me, hunched over their fat bellies. One held up a square device. I could sense their eagerness as their gaze didn't move from mine.

"What happened today?" they asked.

I told them everything. The church. The sentences. How I threw red into Steve's Place, and the devil was inside my dad.

"He was yelling at me very angry…" I said. "I didn't want to kill him, but something kept telling me to."

I rambled until their smug smiles subsided, and they directed me back to the bench.

The agonizing minutes passed by. Eventually, a man in black walked into the room with the yellow sock I left in the blue bin at Steve's Place. He pulled out the slip of paper and read the sentences out loud.

Maybe now they'd understand who I am. Maybe I'd be set free.

But nope. No response.

My words made no difference.

Phony self exposed.

* * *

My mom and sister Karmen arrived. My mom wore a blue jacket and light-colored jeans. I gave her a long and deep hug, feeling sad it was my last time seeing her.

"I love you."

Karmen, who wore black leggings and a black jacket, went to hug me. I backed away—her face heartbroken. I wanted to, but she wore black. When I saw her bright pink shoes, I realized why I couldn't hug her. She was pregnant.

I will return as her child. I could still save humanity.

I felt comforted knowing I'd see my family again. After they left, a man in black escorted me outside where the sky depressed the atmosphere and puddles filled the earth. Crisp water dripped on my skin until I was put in a car by a woman in black—my mom's car nearby.

"I must say I love them once more," I told the woman.

She expressed a heavy sadness—as if, for one second, she felt my pain and, maybe, knew who I was. But my request was denied. The man in black who joined us whispered into her ear and drove us off.

I didn't question why two people escorted me. Nor did I question where we were going. I knew where the roads led.

The cliff on the hill.

As we neared the trailhead, I daydreamed. Rainfall hid the twilight sky. Infrequent sounds of birds and bugs—a steady trickle of water. I'd walk the narrow path of trees and step to the stone's edge.

For one last time in my body, I would smell the air and touch my skin. No one else would be around—just me. With no thought—no feeling—I'd let my body drop. I'd live my death.

A perfect fit for the end of my story.

But we made a wrong turn. We parked at another building.

Do I run from here?

Too bad. The silver rings on my ankles and wrists stopped me.

* * *

The three of us walked into a huge empty room. Lines of chairs faced a massive wooden desk. From a door in the back, a man stepped out and sat at the desk.

He began speaking, but I wasn't listening. I was distracted by the woman. With light, I could see more of her. She was someone I went to college with but a much older version.

Time has flashed forward.

I was attracted to her warm and inviting presence. I imagined us escaping, running off to the cliff on the hill. Maybe we would talk about life on the way up. Maybe we would kiss before the drop.

"Do you understand?" the man at the desk asked, interrupting my fantasy.

I nodded my head in agreement.

I understand what's going to happen.

The three of us left. The woman helped me in the backseat of the car, and we continued driving. However, we were still going the wrong way, picking up speed on the expressway.

How will we escape to the hill now?

Every bump and maneuver of the car made me think we were going to crash. To protect us, I clamped my hands in prayer and pointed my fingertips toward the man driving.

Let us be safe.

I didn't want anyone to die. Just me. But it had to be on the hill.

I felt relieved when we arrived at a garage. The driver brought me into a room with a tall desk and glass walls concealing separate, smaller rooms. Others in black stood around.

Now is the time.

When I looked for the woman, she was nowhere to be found. Instead, those in black forced me into a smaller room that had a massive, obsidian-tinted window on the wall.

Deep into the void, I saw the faint outline of an older woman.

"Have you ever thought about hurting yourself?" she asked through a speaker.

Bang! Bang! Bang! Loud gunshots echoed as I heard screams of terror from the man and woman who brought me.

She shot him.

Blood from the man's head splattered on the wall. I sensed her presence coming to me.

Finally, we're escaping.

But she didn't come. Rather, a man directed me to a silver-coated shower and gave me green pants and a T-shirt to change into. Angst choked my throat as hot water boiled my skin.

I never saw the woman again. I was being mocked.

I can't be in the right place.

I wasn't.

* * *

A man in black forced me down a long, dismal hallway. Dirt smudged its white walls and floors. Lights flickered from above. Crackling bulbs shivered my spine as if we approached something wicked.

I kept my hands in prayer. I stepped to the hall's center, wanting to be symmetrical.

"Get to the right!" the man yelled, pointing his finger in my face.

I jolted sideways, cringing at the motions of my body. I wanted to stop making mistakes.

We arrived at a massive, open space with gated rooms around the perimeter. The man led me to the corner where a few cells were fenced in (shown on page 199).

An extra layer of protection from me.

Another man in black was on the other side of the fence. He brought me in and put me in a small room.

"Go to bed now," he said.

Craaank! The steel door thundered as it closed.

I could barely walk around the room. A silver toilet sat in the corner. On top of a stone bed were a thin green pad and a gray blanket. A white ledge glued to the wall hung above its end. Black marks—some words, some drawings—scribbled its murky cement.

I quivered. I felt used and weak, trembling at the thought of staying here. But all I could do was sleep.

I unraveled the blanket and laid down, covering my shivering body to feel a degree warmer. The stiff bed aggravated my knees and elbows.

I was at rock bottom.

What went wrong?

I was no longer the person I was before. I wasn't someone of hope—someone who inspired insight into the universe with a vision of enhancing the greater good. Instead, humanity was to remain limited—torn by its fragile understanding of mastering the strength in one another.

It was over. My mission was over. I had to let it go.

At least I can still dream.

* * *

I had no dream. In a hot and sudden sweat, my eyes shot open from the scorching lights above my head. Everything smelled like rancid, decaying bodies.

I felt sick. I rushed to the toilet, gripped its sides, and violently threw up. Blood poured out of my mouth like a waterfall—my innards flushed.

Through the door window, a man in black stared at me with a deceiving smile. A slimy bubble tickled my throat, and I shoved my hand in to rip it out.

"Stop doing that!" the man shouted.

He appeared at the door. When I saw a gold star on his shirt, I listened. I dropped my body onto the floor. I looked toward the toilet to see how the blood had vanished.

Holy shit.

I didn't want to move. I didn't know what was happening or what was going to happen.

Vulgar voices began speaking to me. They sounded like gremlins—mischievous creatures from Hell sent to torture me.

"Look how pathetic he is. He's no God. He's weak," the gremlins said. "Worthless. Worthless. Worthless piece of shit."

I wanted to hide my face. I wanted to lie on the bed and curl under the blanket.

Boom, boom, boom! Heavy knocks pounded on the door.

"Get out from under there," the man in black said. "You can't cover yourself during the day."

I listened. I stood and threw the blanket onto the floor. The man yelled at me again.

"Stupid. Stupid. Stupid," the gremlins added. "He can't figure it out."

I put the blanket back on myself. But the man's forceful words—muffled by the obnoxious voices laughing—repeated themselves.

What am I doing wrong?

I went through a series of moving the pad and the blanket on the bed, floor, and back again. I eventually figured it out. The man stopped his outrage when the blanket and pad remained on the bed, and I sat on the floor trembling.

Please, I need a moment to breathe.

I tried to understand how I ended up here. But I could barely hear myself. So many voices penetrated every lobe of my brain. At some point, memories returned.

I remembered what I did to my dad. I remembered wanting to self-sacrifice. I remembered the woman not saving me.

Maybe I'm on the way to Hell.

I feared that thought. Never seeing my family, friends, or the light of day again—I'd rather have been lifeless.

Maybe, I could still do something.

I sat on my knees and squeezed my palms at my chest. I didn't expect my prayers to resolve anything, but I wanted to try.

"I swear I am a good person," I said out loud. "I never meant to do the things I did. Forgive me. I want to see my family again."

On and on, I prayed. On and on, I tried to feel some form of hope.

"Hahaha…you are never leaving," the gremlins said. "No one is saving you."

Please, God, please. Forgive me.

* * *

A circular ball of white, fluffy shreds appeared in the toilet. It was glowing—the silver lining of the transparent water surrounded its sacred holiness.

It's a galaxy—a gift presented from higher beings.

Craaank. The deafening crack of the door startled me.

I snagged the ball and shoved it in my throat, consuming the holiness before they noticed.

"Don't eat that!" a man in black shouted.

Shit, they caught me.

Two men walked into the room and picked me up off the floor. I had no choice but to go with them.

This is it. I'm on my way to Hell.

The next thing I knew, I was in an office. A tan man in a black suit sat behind a desk. A pale woman in a gray suit stood with her arms on his shoulder. Their menacing eyes glared at me as if I were something evil.

"They're going to punish him," the gremlins said. "He's a bad man. Bad man!"

Question after question—I couldn't decipher who was saying what.

"Did you take bath salts?" someone asked.

"I…uh…I don't think so," I responded.

"If you don't say you took bath salts, you won't get out of here," a voice said.

I wanted to leave. I didn't want to go to Hell. With a plea of desperation, I said yes to the bath salts. All of a sudden, I was in the caged-in room, stomach on the green pad.

"She's coming to shoot you," a voice said.

I looked toward the door to see a man in black who appeared to be the brother of Carrie—the girl I was supposed to marry.

Why is he here? Is she coming to complete the task?

I wanted to die so desperately. But when the room quieted and the door creaked open, I shook with nerves.

Tip tap tip tap tip tap. Soft steps neared.

I felt her presence. Her soft lips. Her velvet hair.

"I'm sorry," she said, raising a gun to the back of my skull.

I couldn't maintain composure.

Plop plop plop. My body sprung on the pad's elastic casing.

I couldn't stop shaking. Within a split second, I was in the office again.

"You have to stay still for it to work," the man and woman said. "You don't want to make another mistake."

"I know…I know…" I said, fluttering with fear.

The white blur flashed, and I returned to the pad.

I squeezed my stomach inward. I stared at the cement in front of me. Noticing a thin strand of black hair, I circled my fingers above it and concentrated.

In and out…in and out…in and out, I breathed. My heartbeat slowed. My body unfurled.

Carrie's faint cry returned.

Goodbye…

Bang! The gun shot.

All my thoughts, memories, and connections to the world flashed in my mind and disappeared. For a split second, before everything went dark, I felt happy.

I can finally rest.

Sunken despair.

* * *

After cops arrested me, I thought I was going to Hell, not the booking process for jail.

Fingerprinting. Mugshot. Interview for my statement. Trip to the courthouse where a judge indicted me. I like to think the woman I found comfort in was an officer feeling sympathy, but she may have been a hallucination.

Psychosis, particularly in jail, has changed me. Living has never felt the same, and I don't think it ever will. Unlike growing up and painting Easter eggs with family to symbolize new life—easygoing days of no uncertainty—my existence can now obscure unwillingly.

My identity. My perception. My reality sometimes fritters away into an endless atmosphere, and I have to find ways to keep the puzzle of my life together.

One reason I wrote this book.

There's no question that incarceration exacerbated my illness. Cells were dirty. Guards yelled at me when I broke the rules. I couldn't walk in the hall how I wanted to or use the blanket during the day.

Control was the priority. Not my health and recovery. Initial psychiatric evaluation notes said drugs were to blame.

> *It appears he became psychotic under the influence of drugs and is gradually coming out of it. He is not able to carry on a relevant, coherent conversation. He initially denied having any problems with his father or using drugs. However, he then talked about how he was possessed by Satan. He later on admitted that he has been using marijuana, drinks booze on the weekends, and has used bath salts.*

I'm disgusted they immediately blamed drugs—as if I chose to experience psychosis and that justified punishment. Clearly, their misunderstanding and apathy were present from the start.

After the initial evaluation, I had a crisis therapy session. Throughout this time, I believed I was flashing back and forth between the office and jail cell.

I don't know what the bubble in my throat was. I don't know what I hallucinated when speaking with those in the office who I assume were treatment providers. I imagine the smell of rancid bodies was an olfactory hallucination, and the galaxy was balled up toilet paper.

But I don't really know.

My consciousness was highly distorted. What others saw didn't resemble what was in my mind.

I didn't puke blood. I wasn't shot. I never took bath salts. But was I a criminal? Did I deserve to be in jail—even if I did use bath salts? What would've been the ideal place for me to recover?

Jails cannot be the place for those in a mental health crisis. Yet that's where many go. Nearly a third of people in US jails have at least one diagnosed mental illness. Approximately one-fifth of that third include psychosis.

Therapy was useless due to the severity of my illness. Medication might have helped, but it would take days to get prescribed. Only time would tell if I'd ever escape my reality.

How much worse could I become?

AWOKEN NIGHTMARE

Everything was red—the pad, the toilet, the floor, and the ceiling. Jet black concealed a narrow window at the top of the cell. Dark orange light burned in the corner.

It felt hot and sinister—like something out of a haunted house.

But why is Hell so quiet?

A man in black I'd never seen before sat outside. He was reading a book. When he saw me, a bewildering bolt of energy struck my body.

I jumped up and ran to the door, curious if I could leave. The man smirked as I tried opening it. Although locked, I was a God once.

I could break through.

I stepped to the thick steel, pulled my fist back, and slammed the window with a hard thrust. My attempt only resulted in damaged knuckles and squeals from the asshole on the other side.

"Don't be doing that," he said. "Go to bed."

Fury enraged my clenched fists. The gut-wrenching, chest-splitting idea of forever in Hell made me want to scratch my eyes out and crack my skull on the cement.

What can I do?

I paced back and forth, nervous and shaking. When I saw tiny circles embedded in the orange light, I stared at them. Shades of color rippled throughout, and every time darkness crept from the edge, I shunned it away.

Hope.

I control light.

Hours after protecting the circles, I noticed a silver shelf with a round bolt fixed to the wall. A circle of light formed around it, but it wouldn't enclose completely. So I centered my eyes and stared.

I must bring the sun back—it will light my path out the window.

The more I tried to succeed, the more pressure built on my shoulders. Eventually, the circle lined up perfectly.

I won—I'm victorious.

I hopped on the bed to look out the window. Instead of the sun, a dozen polished stars—giant bulbs—hovered nearby. I was in awe of their soft, delicate beauty. They were much larger than usual.

I must be in the center of space.

Bang! Bang! Bang! Fists slammed on the door.

"Get down and go to bed!" the man in black shouted.

What a fucking prick.

Jesus shouldn't be trapped in Hell.

Yet here I am.

* * *

Burning white light forced my eyes open. It looked like I had been transported to a new cell. Outside the door, a tall man in green stared at me as he talked to a man in black.

"You don't trust him," the gremlins whispered. "You shouldn't trust him."

Does he know who I am?

Behind him was a mass of people—prisoners of Hell—wearing the same green.

Satan is the master of mockery.

The man in black handed me a white container.

"Ooooh, what is that? Don't trust that."

I opened it to see breakfast food. However, the smell of feces engulfed my nose, and I gagged.

"Hahaha, it's shit!" the gremlins uttered. "Eat it! Eat it! Eat that shit!"

I shoved the container back towards the man.

What else were they brewing in Hell's Kitchen?

The voices gave me their most festive ideas—ground-up body parts, sewage sludge. They continued to torment me, convincing me a sniper shot at me. I danced around my cell, dodging the bullets.

They described how Hell took over earth, torturing everyone I knew. Hair-raising sounds and images in my head—fire burning, human mutilation, pools of blood—confirmed their words.

The prisoners glorified Hell's takeover—free to indulge in pure evil. They'd come back and party, praising Satan and me.

I am evil.

At one point, I heard my mom's voice.

"Help me, Cohen. Help me."

"I'm going to rape her," a dark, grisly voice said. "You can't do anything."

Satan.

My stomach curdled—like spoiled meat seeping its foul stench into my heart.

What the fuck.

"Please don't," I pleaded.

But he was right. I couldn't do anything.

Hahaha. Satan laughed while my mom screamed in agony.

I'm sorry, Mom...I'm so sorry.

Guilt rotted every part of my soul. All I could do was succumb to it. I felt more than dead—I was eternally shamed for the most horrific thing to happen to humanity.

The universe is ending, and I let evil win.

* * *

I sat on the green pad to settle my pain. A puny, white dot appeared underneath the skin of my wrist.

What could it be?

"He's the one. He's the one," the gremlins said. "Our Lord has chosen."

An embryo—Satan's child.

I felt repulsed by my own being. I wanted to rip off my skin and melt onto the floor. Throughout my entire journey, I thought I was someone of courage and spirit. But I was wrong. I was nothing but the devil's accessory with the duty of providing an heir to the king of Hell.

Curious about Hell's success on earth, I quickly glanced out the window. My dad's work truck drove on a distant road—a burnt putrid red coated the entire landscape.

Another mockery.

I miss you, Dad.

I refused to move for hours. I didn't want to cause more destruction.

"Someone will come for you," the gremlins said. "Don't move, not even your head!"

Frozen like an ice-cold statue, I desperately held onto the prospect of escaping Hell. But a gloomy shadow coaxed my skin and bones.

No one came. Life was black.

I'm never leaving.

Desolate sorrow.

* * *

Sweating—my skin bled with slimy grease.

What now?

The room was sweltering—coated in a golden color. Two men with gold stars pinned on their black shirts peered in from the door.

"He's our only hope," they said.

The sun.

I felt an electric numbness at my feet. The vibration traveled up my body, sewing a sting with each nerve.

I'm becoming a Sun God.

When the process arrived at my heart, I started to shake—the force wouldn't pass through.

"Stop bouncing," the Sun Gods yelled. "Stop!"

But I couldn't help it. The shocking pain was too much.

"He's been sacrificed, right?" a Sun God asked.

"I've died twice," I said. "Once at the church and once before Hell."

"He should've only been sacrificed once."

Failing at death was sardonic at this point. But then, an apparition emerged nearby.

It's the God of All Things.

I recognized his eyes—filled with tears.

Why is he sad?

As he vanished, I looked up and saw the Twin Towers drawn in the ceiling, crumbling. I recalled a memory from third grade, watching it happen on TV.

That wasn't my fault.

Was humanity the reason evil won?

Is any of this my fault?

Should humanity be responsible for how the world turns out?

"It all started from the beginning," a soft voice interrupted.

I shed my clothes and huddled in a fetal position.

I am the beginning. I am the end.

Without question, I shoved a thumb into my rectum.

"Ahhhhhh!" I belched.

My high-pitched, deafening shriek lit the room in blazing white. The door burst open. The voices choked. Dark figures shuffled in and circled me.

"Heeelp…" I murmured, as they gripped my shoulders and dragged me.

My legs scraped on the floor—my arms dangling like a lifeless doll.

What's next?

* * *

Space travel again. This place felt similar, but it had no window, and outside the door was a tiny square room.

I looked at the floor, spotting an obscure pattern of mismatched colors and lines. Cords of hair, plucks of dirt, and white clumps plastered the motif with a sea of galaxies.

It's the universe. I'm outside the realms of time and space.

Careful not to step on the universe, I walked along the floor's edge and to the door.

"I don't get it. What am I supposed to do here?" I asked.

The man in black pointed to the silver spout on the toilet's tank.

"Drink," he said.

Although cautious, I listened. Clear liquid streamed out of the spigot—cold and crisp; it tasted like heaven. But suddenly, the bubble behind my tongue pulsated, and something inside my stomach tingled.

It's time.

I lay on the green pad to calm myself. However, my throat blocked up, and my chest tightened.

Fuck.

I spread my legs. I squeezed my core. I breathed heavily as my stomach roared.

Stay calm. Stay calm.

Breathing in and out…in and out…I felt like I was about to split open. After minutes of extreme force, I felt the bubble release.

Peeeeeew plonk. The sound of a drop in stomach acid.

No baby.

It must've been destroyed when becoming a Sun God.

I struggled to believe something good happened.

"I want to go home," I said out loud. "I want to see family and friends."

I wanted the nightmare to end so badly—tears streamed down my face.

"We love you, Cohen," the voices of my family said. "We're here for you. You did nothing wrong."

"Can I come home, please?"

"You are home," my dad said.

I pictured it. A quiet place surrounded by trees—light shining through the foliage.

"What do you think little bro? A cabin?"

Yes, a cabin.

Such a peaceful place it would be.

"Cohen, don't ever change the way you are."

My God. Thank you.

A sliver of hope.

* * *

God of All Things appeared outside the door in full form. He stood with a younger bald man who had knife-like tattoos.

Satan.

Satan wore the same gold star as the God of All Things. His pitch-black eyes bled with angry tears.

Why is he upset? Wouldn't he have wanted Hell to take over?

Perhaps he knew how critical balance was to live.

He opened the door and demanded I go with him. I followed—hands in prayer—to an area with two rooms on opposite sides.

The door on the left was open. I glanced in, my eyes meeting a man who looked oddly familiar. He wore the same clothes as me, but his smile made me feel like he knew something I didn't.

Satan led me to the other room. Through a large window, I saw an older version of Carrie. Her voice was muffled—I couldn't understand. But I imagined her future self appeared to tell me it was too late to be together.

I didn't care.

Who's the man in the other room?

As Satan walked me back, I pictured every detail of him. His hair, eyes, and cheekbones—each feature resembled someone I felt very connected to yet barely knew.

Who is he?

I rested my eyes and thought about the beginning—the start of the path that led me to Hell. I thought about the professor and our first meeting. I thought about my sentences.

Everything felt crystal clear. But something of critical value was missing.

What is it?

Temporary darkness made me realize the blinding light.

Arthur.

A. R.—the lanky man I met in the hospital. A. R.—the man who mainly talked to the baby angels but snagged my attention. A. R.—the man I wrote the sentence in the Bible for.

A. R.—he was the man in that room.

He knew I was the prophet. He knew what to say to get my ear and voice. I gave him the secret of the universe, and he used it against me.

How didn't I realize this before?

He was the reason everything became fucked up.

But why is he here—in the same position as me?

I recalled the Twin Towers—how humanity must take responsibility for the world. I recalled the God of All Things telling me not to change. I recalled him and Satan in the same room and the importance of balance.

The Law of the Universe has been judging our fate.

They knew everything about me. They knew everything about everything.

How could one man alter the universe?

I wasn't in Hell. I couldn't control the sun and planets. I wasn't Jesus.

I was duped—mind controlled by A. R.

What made me think I could manipulate the Universe?

I was a single human. Someone who once loved to run and study in college. Someone whose family and friends cared for him.

Someone with a name—Cohen.

Cohen.

Cohen.

What have you been doing?

Stop.

Stop thinking. Stop doing.

Let go.

Feel. Feel the moment.

Release the tension.

My body—my mind—they eased.

They melted—exhausted. Tired.

Sleep.

Ready for sleep.

Sleep now.

Covered with the blanket—the cold air cut.

My bones warmed.

My head steadied.

My soul faded.

I took one last look at the floor.

How absurd.

Mending reality.

* * *

The light of day and dark of night overwhelmed me. I didn't know where I was. But now, I know I spent most of my time in one cell. When I screamed, they transferred me to solitary confinement.

I could never imagine the terror of psychosis in jail until I lived through it. Everyone should be outraged at this treatment because I'm not alone. I'm just privileged to have survived.

In 2021, Joshua McLemore's death was captured on video. With severe psychosis, an Indiana jail trapped him in solitary confinement for three weeks.

Officers pinned his naked body against a windowless cell. He licked the wall and floor—soon dirty with feces and gunk. He screamed and tore apart a white Styrofoam container.

For reasons we'll never know, Joshua didn't eat until he was skin and bones. Images reminding me of emaciated victims I'd see studying the Holocaust in the tenth grade.

This could have been me.

I feel twisted at that thought. Dying alone. Cold. Sick. Tormented by a reality breaking the realm of comprehension.

It's sad. It's fucking sad what happened to Joshua.

At this point, my severe psychosis lasted for two weeks with five days in jail. Who knows what would've happened if I had gone to jail sooner.

Progress notes describe my situation.

> *He is on the edge of his bunk, eyes are staring. Writer informed him he was in the Steuben County Jail. He did not know where he was. He appears to be responding to internal stimuli but is unable to say what they are. He was encouraged to eat properly. He shook his head that he would try. Client does not appear to be safe to be removed from constant watch* [twenty-four-hour watch because of suicide risk].

I couldn't stomach food, thinking it was disguised shit. I struggled to break away from command hallucinations—what I heard as the gremlins speaking to me. I couldn't recognize the men in black as jail guards or the men in green as inmates. Even the simple, dirty floor made me believe I was seeing the universe.

Years later, in New York City's Metropolitan Museum of Art, I saw Cy Twombly's painting *Dutch Interior*. Its abstract scribbles and smears reminded me of the floor. A distortion of reality that struck me in the gut.

No one knew if or when I would return from psychosis. But where was I to go? What would've helped? Could my torment have been avoided if my mental health had been supported long before jail?

What would it take for society to prioritize mental health—to make its support an essential part of our culture that is encouraged, accessible, and viable?

I was comforted by my family's voices and connection to God of All Things. When Satan's baby was destroyed, and the Twin Towers appeared, I began wondering if I truly ended the universe.

With Arthur, I questioned my entire experience. He was never in that jail. But his presence—and everything else that shifted my perception—tipped the delusional story I was stuck in. I started to become aware of who I was and where I was.

Was my mind healing? Could I finally stop worrying and relax?

Was I on the road to recovery?

Sentences posted on Facebook

Satan: Hahahahaha
Dieu: Tu ris pour quoi?
Satan: Je me moque de toi
Dieu: Pourquoi?
Satan: Donc tu veux dire que tu
aimes tes
enfants et qu'eux aussi

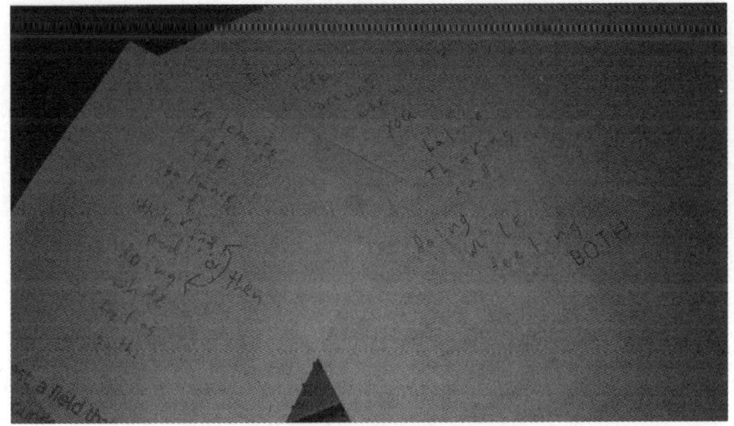

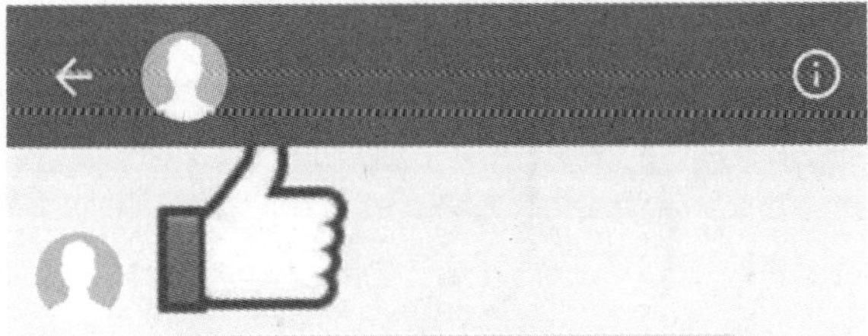

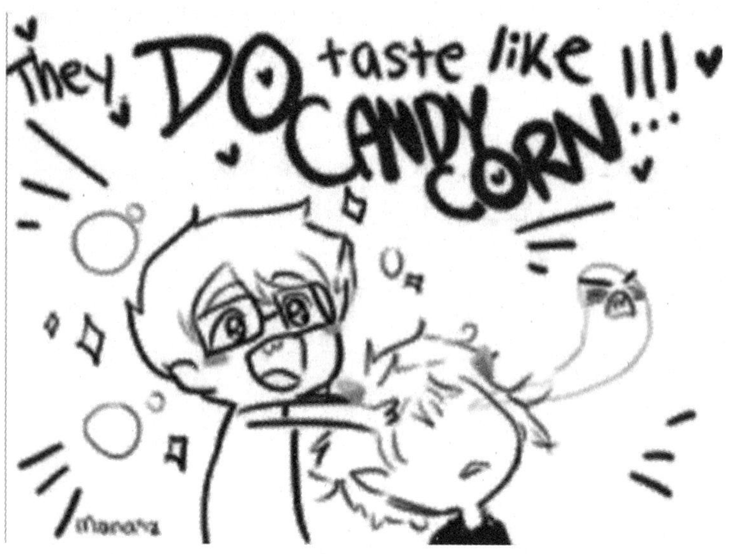

The signs on Facebook that led to Cohen attacking Dad

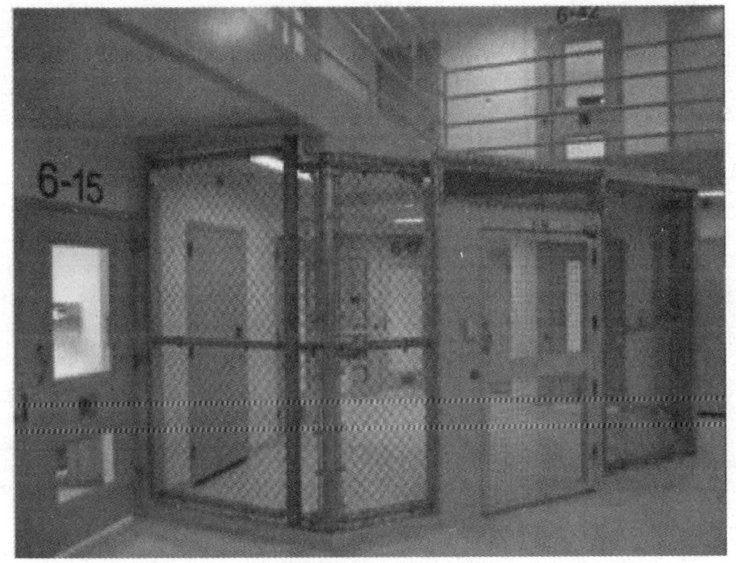

The fenced in jail cell

PART IV

REALITY REBORN

I slept peacefully for hours. I walked on the floor without fear of stepping on the universe. I drank as much water as I could. Voices came, but I didn't respond.

When given my next meal, I scooped corn into my mouth. It smelled and tasted like actual shit.

"Don't eat it if you're going to puke," a man in black said.

I was determined, however. I took a slow breath, drank more water, and tried again. Somehow, it now tasted like regular, shitty corn.

What changed?

While I devoured the entire meal—unsure of when I last ate—the man in black approached the cell.

"You used to be a pretty fast runner, huh?" he asked.

How does he know…

"Another guard here went to high school with you," he added.

Oh…okay…that's okay.

"I used to love running," I said.

"What's your fastest mile?"

"I was known for the 5K…but I think my mile was 4:20."

"That's awesome, man. My friend said you were amazing."

Look at me now.

In a cell with nowhere to go, I didn't know how much time passed. But I was getting tired of looking at the walls. When a guard offered me a book, I was quick to accept.

The book was about an architect from a poor rural town who traveled to a distant city and learned how to build sustainable buildings. Her goal was to advance the homes in her community, but she was absorbed by wealth, power, and fame. After misery for some time, she returned—embraced by those who raised her whether or not she improved their homes.

"Wow, he's reading," the guard whispered to himself.

I felt connected to the story. I related to the character, and the narrative controlled my thoughts. Sometimes, however, the words on the pages would change. I'd stop to sleep and then read a few pages back to see different words.

Fascinating.

I acknowledged the uncertainty. I didn't let it distract me from finishing the book. Eventually, I succeeded.

I made it to the resolution.

* * *

A guard unlocked the door and directed me to follow him. I stayed on the right side of the hallway. Instead of putting my hands in prayer, I gripped my book. We stepped into a large room with fenced-in cells in the corner.

I've been here before.

The air was silent and still. The guard led me to the corner; dozens of people in green stared at me as if I were a mythical creature. At the fence was the man in black who resembled the God of All Things. But at that point, he looked like a typical man.

Someone like my dad. Balding hair. Fat belly. Weariness from a hard day's work.

He's just a guard doing his job.

The cell colors were soft and bland—nothing stood out. I was so used to seeing the toilet, sleeping pad, and blanket that the familiarity was somewhat calming. When I glanced towards the window, I couldn't believe my eyes.

Blue sky!

I jumped on the bed to see more, quickly looking at the guard, fearing he'd yell at me.

"Please step down," he patiently asked.

"One minute...please."

He agreed.

I was captivated by an extraordinary landscape of grass, trees, sidewalks, and brick buildings. Light poles had big round bulbs at their top. Birds flew, and leaves swirled in the wind.

My eyes quivered. The beauty was unlike anything I'd seen before.

What a miracle life is. What a miracle.

It was official. Hell, never took over earth.

I was safe. My family was safe.

Everyone is safe.

Wish come true.

* * *

The guard handed me a Styrofoam container of food. Inside was a small cup of purple liquid.

"It's grape juice," he said.

My hands shook as I picked it up to drink. Drops of the sweet, sticky liquid splattered onto the floor. I wanted what was happening to be real life so badly. But fear of the unknown continued to obstruct my perception.

Am I really not in Hell?

The guard looked disappointed.

"I'm sorry," I said.

"It's okay."

I heard a shower running in the distance.

"Can I take a shower?" I asked.

I hadn't bathed in a long time.

"I'll make you a deal. If you clean the grape juice, I'll let you shower," he said.

I could do that.

He gave me a bottle and towel. I sprayed and scrubbed, watching the floor morph from purple-spotted to clear white.

Fascinating.

"Do you have clean clothes?" he asked.

I didn't have to say anything for him to know the answer.

"I figured. On me."

He gave me a fresh pair of pants, a shirt, and underwear. He let me out of the cell, pointing to the shower.

"Thank you so much," I said.

* * *

The shower was warm and calming. Water soaked my hair. Soap smoothed my skin. I had been repulsed by my body for so long, but now, I was free from dirt and grime. It felt as though I was slowly regaining control of myself.

What now?

Hour by hour, I sat in the cell. The guards changed. The day dimmed. Lines of shadow through the window curved on the walls.

The next meal arrived, and the guard let me out of the cell and its fenced-in area. In the large common area, men—the other inmates—lined up behind a cart stacked with brown containers.

I stepped in the back, peering over their shoulders to see what it was. When I noticed a single blue container at the bottom, I quickly moved to get it. Everyone gasped.

"He thinks he's special!" someone shouted.

I withdrew, confused and worried.

"I'll get it for you," the guard at my cell said, directing me back.

He gave me the brown container, but I was unsure how to manage it. It was much larger than the Styrofoam one.

"You place it there and sit at the end of the bed," he said, pointing at the white ledge.

Ah, okay.

My hunger was intense. I devoured the hot dogs, creamed corn, bread, and milk—everything tasted like heaven. Not a single idea or worry passed through my mind.

After I finished the meal, I sat back and smiled.

I'm not in Hell.

* * *

The day I discovered I was in jail was a day of many realizations.

I am Cohen.

I was not the prophet. I was not a God who took control of the universe and destroyed humanity. Hell wasn't ravaging earth, and Satan didn't rape my mom or implant a baby in me.

The world was the same as it had always been.

Nothing changed except for me.

I processed everything immediately. The hallucinations, bizarre thoughts, and delusional stories—I was in awe of what happened and had to make sense of it. Thankfully, I wasn't alone.

"Do you know where you are, and why you're here?" the psychiatrist asked.

"Yes, I'm in jail because I attacked my father."

She was so happy I was doing better. But I was worried—really worried.

I faced two felonies. One was a second-degree assault for what happened with my dad. The other was third-degree criminal mischief when I broke the window at Steve's Place. That meant potentially a decade in prison.

How could I live with that?

"Why can't I go somewhere else?" I said. "I'm feeling better."

"Cohen," she said, eyes locked onto mine. "You are in a very serious situation."

"But I couldn't control what I did to my dad."

"I know...but you tried to give birth in the jail cell."

My eyes fell. My shoulders dropped. I flashbacked to the moment—my legs bent up as I squeezed and pushed. I must've looked ridiculous. Nothing would come out of my stomach because I couldn't give birth.

How the fuck could I think that?

"I had a young man in a similar situation as you, and he was able to move on," she added. "If you do everything right—follow the rules and stick to the plan—you might be able to leave and have a promising future."

Her words smacked me in the face. I had to listen if I was going to get out of jail.

I have to listen.

"I'm prescribing you Zyprexa, an antipsychotic. Take it once a night before bedtime."

"Will do," I said without question.

I wanted all the help I could get.

I want to stay healthy.

* * *

The jail moved me into a new cell shortly after I met with the psychiatrist. One with access to a general population area. This new cell block had inmate workers, meaning most would be gone throughout the day. The space would be quieter—more ideal for recovery.

I settled into my new cell with barely any possessions. When I stepped outside my cell, an inmate I never met approached me.

"What'd you do to get in here?" he asked.

"I…uh…was in a fight with my dad…" I replied.

"Oh, you were the guy who bit his dad's ear off?"

How?! How does he know?

Before I could ask, he said his girlfriend told him how someone went crazy and bit their dad's ear off.

"You made the news, dude."

Part of me was relieved. His knowing wasn't a sign from the universe. He didn't have a cosmic connection to my story. He had just heard about it secondhand through local news. But I was worried about what others thought of me.

My friends, my family…does everyone hate me? Am I an evil monster?

As afraid as I was, I couldn't do anything. I was in jail. I wasn't ready to discuss my feelings with a stranger. So I kept them inside, waiting to meet with the psychiatrist again.

* * *

I familiarized myself with the new cell block. Everything was cold steel—bleak colors of white and pastel pink. A staircase led to a balcony where more cells were located.

The general population area included a TV, games, tables, and a tall desk where a guard sat twenty-four-seven-days-a-week. Looping the perimeter, I had enough distance to walk maybe fifty meters.

Jail made the hospital look like paradise.

A half-dozen inmates stood around. A few watched a news report of a town flood. I joined, seeing people trek through several feet of water while holding stuff above their heads.

"Some prophet," I heard a man nearby say. "He wasn't going to save anyone."

Did I cause the flood?

It didn't make sense. I was not the prophet. The world was not ending.

Did someone actually say that?

I recalled the psychiatrist revealing my delusional thoughts and behavior. I recalled what put me in jail—my experience in jail.

No way.

I continued looping the perimeter. I saw an elderly man stumbling, talking gibberish like he was drunk. A guard and an inmate laughed as he couldn't find the toilet to take a shit.

"Fuck. Now someone's gotta clean that up," the guard said.

Is that what I looked like?

I felt sad for him. He needed a lot more support than what jail could give.

Next, I stumbled upon payphones glued to the wall. I picked one up, wanting to call my dad. However, I had no money to dial.

"Niii…ce…trrr…y…," I heard a voice say as I hung up.

It began as a typical pitch of a man's voice but quickly became deep and demon-like. It was also the same voice as the inmate I met, yet he was standing on the other side of the room.

An auditory hallucination.

I started to feel more uncertain about what my mind turned into.

I need help in every possible way.

The will to be well.

* * *

Time was essential to healing. After realizing where I was, I accepted my mental illness and began taking steps to manage my wellness. Most importantly, I wanted treatment—I wanted to be healthy.

It's not easy to accept mental illness. Again, no one wants to be ill. I see the stigma and lack of understanding of mental health all the time. Sadly, my situation helped me.

The pain with my father. The misery of psychosis. The potential of jail for years—which still angers me today. I'm not surprised how I responded to treatment this time. I just wish I didn't have to get to such a dark place to change.

Recovery is a process of change that improves an individual's health and wellness. From the psychiatric progress notes, I was improving.

> *Inmate came into session stating he has been doing better this week. He has been, reportedly,*

> *sleeping, eating, and drinking well. Inmate's mood appeared mildly anxious and depressed. He continues to show signs of delusional thinking.*

I'm so happy I finally ate, drank, and slept regularly. Although symptom severity decreased, they were still present. Just like acceptance and physiological needs, awareness and coping skills were critical for my recovery.

When I heard the statement regarding the flood on the TV, I identified the hallucination and how my brief prophetic thoughts were delusional. I coped by continuing my perimeter walk and reflecting on therapy. I did the same after I heard the voice when hanging up the payphone.

These initial steps to care for my health helped me get where I am now. With my first experience of severe psychosis occurring throughout one month, I began learning how to manage it fairly quickly. Something I am indebted to as I now know how essential early intervention is to effective recovery.

But again, these are only lasting effects of the miracle that gave my future hope. If it wasn't for the support from those I interacted with in jail, I don't know if I would be where I am now either.

A guard was ready to offer me a book—surprised when I read. A guard let me look out the window although it broke the rules. A guard guided me in cleaning the grape juice and invested his own money, so I could have clean clothes. I even remember in the throes of psychosis, a guard writing water on a cup in hopes I would finally drink.

These small acts of kindness gave me glimmers of hope when I had nothing else. I will always be grateful for them.

Was it possible for me not to accept the illness—maybe if I faced a minor crime or moderately severe psychosis? What if the guards never showed care or a psychiatrist wasn't available—would I have started the recovery process effectively? What if I claimed to be the Prophet again—would I have returned to solitary confinement and died like Joshua McLemore?

I was taking my health seriously. But I still had a long way to go. The chains—both invisible and evident—remained.

When would I be released?

SEEKING SUPPORT

Time in jail blurred. I didn't pay attention to the date or concern myself with missing college graduation. Instead, I walked the perimeter of the cell block every day.

"Not the same as a track, huh?" the guard from my high school said.

"Nope," I said, moving forward.

I did push-ups in the corner. I slept as soon as possible—meds knocked me out each night.

On the table in my cell, I lined up photos from the mail. Pictures with friends and family. Pictures of my mullet and scene-kid days. I wasn't sure whether to laugh or cry.

I kept a stack of letters in close company, reading them every day (shown on page 266-268).

"Hi bud! I love you. You mean everything to me. You will need to be patient and do what doctors say. We will get through this," my dad wrote, hiding his name from the letter. "The state will not allow Gram and I to have any contact with you, so your mom will communicate between you and me. We are here to help."

"Hey Brother! I think about you every day," Karmen wrote. "I truly hope you're given the help and tools you need to move on and live that happy, healthy, successful life you've worked so hard for."

"I've been thinking about you a lot," Lindsay wrote. "The conditions you're in; the cold floor, bare walls, and minimal windows. I love you babiest brother. You had one life going for you, you can find another."

"I understand you are disappointed with how your running career went at Geneseo," Rich, a high-school coach, wrote. "Running is often filled with more disappointments than successes. I am pulling for you! A lot of people are."

"I am so sorry for you being in jail since I know you are such a good person," Finn's mom wrote. "You were one of the few people that took initiative to work for the kids in Kenya. KNOW that we are not judging you for these last events. We know what you are made of."

"You have a marathon ahead of you," Finn's dad wrote. "But we're here for you."

I wanted to call my dad. But I couldn't due to the state's restraining order.

Does he hate me? Will he ever forgive me?

The uncertainty tormented me—an enduring shame induced by psychosis.

Maybe I deserve to be here.

My brain may have been healthy, but I wasn't well. I was still in hell.

* * *

Buzzz...click. The sound of leaving the cell block was exciting news.

A guard directed me through the hallway and to the back of a line. I waited anxiously, peering over the men to see a large group of people on the other side of a window. The visitors had to wait until the inmates sat.

Once let in, I saw Finn's smile. He looked nervous. The visitor's space was cold and bleak, and the harsh voices of the guards echoed the tension in the room.

I was nervous too.

What did he think of me?

The room livened up as the guards let the visitors in. Hugs, laughter, and the vibrant voices of the inmates and their loved ones brightened the space.

Finn sat on the other side of the table where a short divider separated us.

"Your dad misses you," he said. "He wishes he could talk to you."

My throat loosened slightly.

"Maybe this would make us closer," I said.

Finn was perplexed. I was too.

What did that mean?

Our conversation quickly turned conventional. He talked about his music and how he missed playing with me. He asked me what I could do in jail and how the food was.

"I'm always hungry, man. I starved myself. Some inmates sneak me extra food though."

He told me about my name in the local news (shown on page 270).

"Whatever happens, man, you have many people supporting you," he said. "Those articles don't mean shit."

"I feel horrible. What are people saying about me?"

"It doesn't matter. What's important is you getting out of here."

I wanted to believe him. Yet I feared the worst.

Other loved ones visited me, including my mom and Casie. Every visit I could have was booked up.

Where would I be if it wasn't for them?

People were still cheering for me.

* * *

My mom sent me money to buy items through the jail commissary. A kiosk in the cell block allowed inmates to purchase deodorant, candy bars, office supplies, and so forth. Two dollars was more than I'd ever spent for instant ramen noodles, but everything was expensive. I had to use money wisely.

After buying toiletries and snacks, I bought a writing pad and pen. I had an idea for a movie and plenty of time to write it.

With a combination of the detective and horror genres, The Devil Caught My Breath followed a young man wrongly convicted of a crime. The opening scene would show him in his cell, writing a statement in a notebook.

"Millions praise the LORD every day, but what makes us believe in God? Faith in something good—some way to think everyone can be happy? What do you really see in reality with so much sin and evil? I must ask, do you believe in the Devil?"

The plot would thicken as something dark would slip through the floor's cracks and consume him. He'd have to find a way to overcome his situation and save himself.

I had no plan for the movie. Writing was a simple coping strategy that eased my boredom. But the inmates were intrigued. I had gotten to know them throughout the days.

We played chess. We made Chi Chi—a potluck of ramen, chips, and whatever else we could put into a bag and cook with hot water. We talked about our lives outside of jail.

I wasn't comfortable sharing my screenplay, but I was willing to share my story—the true story.

* * *

I received transcripts of the statements my grandma, my dad, and I made to the police from my arrest. They painted the grim reality of the incident.

"When I got home Cohen seemed fine," my dad stated. "We were telling him he had to go to the hospital. He then became agitated, repeating, 'This isn't how it is supposed to work,' and 'I need to kill you to save everybody else.'

I was still on the phone with Johanna [Mom], and I told her to call 911. I immediately tried to grab the knife. We wrestled for a while, but he got away from me. I tried talking him down for a few seconds and then realized I had to leave."

I was too ashamed to share the transcripts from my dad and grandma, but I let the inmates read mine.

"I went to the church through the left, red door," I stated. "I finished praying, then drove to Steve's Place in my green Subaru. I wanted to get rid of everything red because it was dangerous. I threw a yellow sock into a blue container, and inside it was a note.

Eventually, my dad came home wearing all black, and I did not like all that black. He was yelling at me, very angry. I took the knife and paced around, and the messages in my phone told me I had to kill my father now. I wasn't trying to actually kill him; I thought I had to for the sake of us. I was hoping he could forgive me."

I didn't feel judged or hated. Instead, the inmates were sad about my situation.

"Chewy doesn't belong here!" one inmate shouted at the guards.

They gave me the nickname Chewy because of what I did to my dad's ear. I wasn't offended. I felt welcomed, mainly when the transcripts made me think my freedom wouldn't come anytime soon.

* * *

I listened to the inmates' stories as much as I could. One young man told me he'd been in and out of jail because of theft.

"I'm half retarded, dude. I can't make it out there," he said. "No one will hire me, so I steal."

I wanted to know more.

Jail isn't working for him.

Another man said he was in a bar fight. As he ruffled through a stack of legal papers, I saw the other man's bloody face.

"I overreacted…but they tryin' to put me away for years though he's fine?" he said. "Public defenders can't do shit… gotta be something I can do."

His motivation to make his case was inspiring.

Should I be doing that?

Another man was in prison for two decades. He killed someone in his teens, referencing gang violence, difficult childhood, and youthful stupidity.

"I was finally free. But then, at a buddy's place, cops came in and busted him for weed," he said. "They picked me up too…for my past. I wasn't even smoking, but here I am, about to return to prison for the rest of my life."

Tears filled his eyes as he described his guilt and remorse—I felt it. I was so sad for him.

"If you get out, man, cherish it."

I took his words to heart.

I could still be free.

* * *

Week after week, my fate swelled within me like a potential flood after a thunderstorm. Eventually, my court hearing arrived.

I had met with a public defender a few times. He instructed the process and a plea bargain, which included probation and required treatment. But I was at the whims of the legal process—far too nervous to fully grasp.

The first thing I noticed when leaving jail was that, for the entire time, I had been in the town I was born in.

The town where my life began...would it end here too?

The drive was lovely. Spring was in full bloom—bright green grass, sunny blue sky. Everything shimmered with vibrancy. It felt as if I was seeing the world for the first time.

I recalled my experience of psychosis. The glaring colors. The messages on street signs. It felt a little too familiar.

I then recognized who was driving.

Satan. How ironic.

He was just another guard of the jail. Someone with a wife and kids. Someone who was being kind to me.

"I've never been to court," I said. "What if I mess up?"

"You'll do fine, kid. And if it goes well, I hope you turn your life around."

* * *

At the courthouse, the guard brought me directly into the courtroom where dozens of citizens sat. The space was quiet and dry, and no one looked happy. Sitting on a bench in the front corner—a holding area—I was visible to everyone.

How special am I to have front-row seating?

One by one, people spoke to the judge. I waited my turn, feeling like another person who received a traffic ticket. My case was far more serious, however, and others knew it—apparent by my jail uniform and jingling cuffs.

I scanned the crowd to see Casie and my mom. We smiled. I had a mixture of excitement to see them and shame for how I was displayed.

I looked like a criminal. I felt like a criminal.

I guess I am a criminal.

When the judge called my name, I froze at the podium. Head still. Eyes forward. The fear of being sentenced for years reminded me of psychosis.

I breathed deeply, trying to relax as I would in a race. But this finish line was different. It was a make-or-break moment in my life.

Please, God, help me get through this.

A woman in black—the district attorney—spoke with the judge about me and the incident. I couldn't hear what was said.

What if I'm not set free? How can I continue my life? Why did this have to happen?

When the judge met his eyes with mine, I stopped thinking. He listed my conditions—probation, conditional discharge, and mandatory treatment.

"Do you understand what you must do and agree to the terms?" the judge asked.

It felt like a movie moment—time was in slow motion, and I was at the center of everything.

"Yes, sir," I said, squeezing my hands together. "Yes, sir."

"We do not see Mr. Miles-Rath as a danger to the community. The plea deal reflects this. The defendant may leave now."

Is it over?

The guard led me to a table near the courthouse exit—my hands shaking. Every second felt like an eternity. Casie walked out of the hall and sat next to me.

"What's going on?" I asked, surprised she could approach me.

"It looks good," she said.

I began to relax, imagining what to do if I could leave.

Go hiking? Visit friends? Eat a big meal?

After a few minutes, my mom stepped out of the hall—her face glowing. The guard followed and uncuffed my arms and legs.

I quickly stood up—a sudden spring in my step. It felt like I had just won the most important race of my life.

I am free.

* * *

I remained calm as we walked to the exit. The moment I stepped outside, I paused.

Hooo...ahhh... I inhaled a deep breath, looking up at the sky.

White fluffy clouds intertwined with the color blue—a sweetened treat for my eyes. The wind brushed against my skin, cooling sweat from my sticky forehead.

I couldn't help but smile. I was ready. I was ready for a new start—a new me.

As we walked toward my mom's car, my dad stood nearby.

Oh my God, how is he here!?

I felt nervous approaching him. His eyes were wide and hesitant. He wore his usual jeans and a light rain jacket.

I spotted the scar on his ear—a small chunk of his lobe missing—and quickly looked away.

"I'm sorry, Dad. I never meant for this."

Not a second later, he leaned in for a hug. A giant squeeze of relief—of warmth and comfort.

"Don't worry about it, son. I love you."

I smiled.

"How are you here?" I asked.

"I wanted to see you—the restraining order will be off soon."

My smile grew.

"You'll live at your mom's for a while, but I'll see you soon."

I understood. I felt so grateful that he even wanted to see me.

He still cares for me.

* * *

My mom drove Casie and me away—my dad waving until he disappeared. I sat back, seeing love in their eyes, and flipped on the car radio—harmonies I missed for so long.

The road home was familiar. I saw where I went to school and had my first kiss. We passed dirt pathways I once ran or rode my bike as a child.

I felt relaxed, watching grass fields and trees pass by. Surrounding hills were gentle and smooth—they always had been.

I am home.

Healthy and free.

* * *

I was desperate for help. I wanted to know people could still care for me—that I could be forgiven and have a future worth living.

It's hard for me to describe how impactful the letters and visits from family and friends were. I truly believed others thought I was a monster—still do, sometimes. But they proved to me I wasn't alone. I was still loved. And I'm blessed to have them in my life.

Even the inmates. Their support revealed to me how empathy and care can come from anyone—judgment would've only added barriers to how we treated each other.

During the final session with my psychiatrist, my mental health improved significantly.

> *Writing is a coping skill for the inmate. He presents as lucid and has been reported to be compliant with staff. He has been eating and drinking well. The focus of the session was on accepting how this will impact his life.*

Focusing on acceptance in therapy and being vulnerable supported wellness. I shared my police statement with the inmates. I talked about my psychosis with the psychiatrist. I was open, honest, and transparent in any way I could be.

What if my family and friends didn't write letters or visit me? What if the inmates didn't care, or what if they mistreated me? What if mental illness continued to have a significant impact, making it difficult for others to help—especially my father?

Recovery is more effective with a supportive community. Healthy relationships, viable treatment, and other protective factors improved my recovery process.

I'll never forget the tremendous relief I felt when seeing my father outside the courthouse. To this day, when thinking about how close he was to losing his life, I comfort myself with all that we have shared.

Slow-dancing in the living room. Driving hours for Philly cheesesteaks. Our haunted house tradition. I would've felt anguished by guilt and disgrace if he never talked to me again.

Although I was free from jail, I was still afraid of what was next. Many consequences, challenges, and obstacles remained.

Where would I go? What would I do?

Could I return to my life before the crisis?

RECOVERY PROGRESS

I was in jail for thirty days. When released, the court dismissed the assault charge and reduced the criminal mischief charge to a misdemeanor. They put me on temporary probation with a year-long conditional discharge. Therefore, I could not break the law, or I risked the charges returning.

I had to pay the owners of Steve's Place four hundred dollars for the broken window. I was required to complete a substance misuse program at the Council on Alcohol and Substance Abuse (CASA) center. I had to see a mental health counselor, a substance misuse counselor, and a psychiatric nurse practitioner every week until they determined I was fit to stop.

For the next year, my life revolved around rehabilitation.

My mom still lived in Dansville, New York. Fortunately, her apartment in the village was an ideal location for me to access a job and treatment.

My dad sold my car thinking I might not be released. So, I had to walk everywhere. I had to walk to CASA. I had to walk to Burger King where I cooked part-time. I had to avoid smoking pot and drinking booze.

I had to do what I had to do to get my life back.

* * *

Therapy was a blessing. I was vulnerable and honest about everything.

I described my upbringing—split family and dysfunctional dynamics. I talked about the pressures of attending college. I discussed my running aspirations, the rise and fall of my college experience, and my last cross-country race—my need to party to feel okay.

I quit a sport I loved. I let go of a girl I loved. I stopped caring about academics.

I never sought help.

I described my illness. My obsession with screenplay writing. My theory. My hospitalizations and resentment of treatment. How I attacked my dad with a knife and went to jail.

"I thought the world depended on me," I said. "I thought I killed everyone, and was sent to Hell where I had to give birth to Satan's child."

"That sounds traumatic," my psychiatric nurse replied. "I can't imagine what that experience was like and how difficult it is to overcome."

Not once did I feel judged or shamed. No generalizations or assumptions were made such as not being able to get better or being spontaneously violent. Instead, therapy helped, even when I continued to face symptoms.

One time, I was at dinner when a song in the restaurant caught my attention.

"It wasn't like how words describe a scenario or how one can interpret something as a sign from God," I said. "But it felt more like a message from forces beyond making me believe something I didn't want to—like I was on the mission again."

"How'd you handle it?" my psychiatric nurse asked.

"I took deep breaths. I focused on dinner. I made a mental note, so I could discuss it with you. I didn't have any other bizarre experience that day so, overall, I felt okay."

"It can be difficult to identify a symptom like that. But processing them as they happen helps. Maybe you could've talked to a family member or friend, so you didn't have to wait. You can call me anytime, especially if symptoms become overwhelming."

Another time, I was driving on the thruway with my dad when a black truck appeared behind us.

"The road was empty until I looked in the rearview mirror. I ignored it at first, but when I looked in the mirror again, the truck was gone."

"How'd that make you feel?" the psychiatric nurse asked.

"Paranoid. I didn't know if it was a hallucination or not."

"It may have been. Or, you might've not seen the truck coming, and it drove off an exit. Fear of psychosis may be having an impact. But as long as you maintain the awareness like you have been, managing any feeling or potential symptom is achievable."

That makes sense.

Challenges to my health, including symptoms, didn't stop. They were just less severe.

* * *

I continued meds since jail. Adjusting my brain's chemicals helped create a space for me to learn how to manage my mental health. However, they weren't entirely beneficial.

I wanted to feel inspired. I wanted to be creative. I wanted energy. But meds restrained my ability to—they were meant to.

I often felt drowsy, gaining weight as I'd stuff my face with discounted Burger King. Unlike the campus restaurant where

I interacted with customers, I was stuck in a greasy kitchen, making burgers according to a screen.

The mile to work was the worst. I trekked the sidewalks in my musty uniform four days a week—morning and night. I'd feel empty, sluggish, and soulless.

I had once been able to run seventy miles a week.

Now look at me, struggling to walk a mile.

I wondered what people thought about me as they drove by.

Do they recognize me?

I used to be in the local news all the time.

"Miles-Rath runs away with yearly awards," they said.

Now, my name had a different tone.

"Troopers say twenty-two-year-old Cohen Miles-Rath attacked his father with a kitchen knife and bit off a chunk of his earlobe."

Facebook comments on the news articles proved to me how people felt.

"He must be related to Mike Tyson!" Janel said.

"You disgusting little punk! I hope your dad cuts you out of his life forever!" Nancy said.

"Another nut," Chris said.

Some people told me how they felt directly.

"You're a crazy lunatic who deserves to stay in jail," someone said.

"Are you going to kill me?" another asked.

I wasn't proud of myself. But I pushed through. I had some support when I posted on my Facebook that I was healthy and free.

"Glad to hear you're out," Will said.

"So happy for ya, Co! You know where you have a friend," Mike said.

"Glad to know you're doing well," Brendan said. "Your GXC/GTF family will always be here for you!"

Some college friends visited me, having breakfast at a local diner and hiking at nearby state park. Conversations focused on memories of our college years and what they were doing since graduation.

Coach Dan and I had lunch together once. I felt grateful to see him as he told me about his up-and-coming athletes.

"Let's stay in touch," he said.

* * *

My nurse practitioner said we could try decreasing the dosage of meds. I trusted him. I wouldn't do anything unless a mental health professional said I could.

The plan was to reduce the milligrams by two and a half every three months. It would take one year to be off meds completely. However, it depended on my reaction.

"If symptoms become unmanageable, we'll have to up the dosage again," he said. "But if we have no significant impact on your day-to-day, I don't see why we can't continue decreasing it. You just have to be honest with me."

"I will," I said. "Trust me, I don't want my symptoms to worsen again."

Bit by bit, the medication's weight lifted off my shoulders. Bit by bit, my mind felt freer to think. Bit by bit, symptoms returned. However, I did my best to recognize them and report back to my treatment team.

Initially, avoiding substance use was difficult, especially as alcohol temporarily relieved my lethargic feelings from the meds. On a couple of occasions, I snuck a few drinks. If I timed it right, CASA's weekly drug tests would never catch me, and they didn't.

One night was with Cody. After some beers loosened us, we sat on the stoop at my mom's and had a heart-to-heart.

"You're the golden child, little bro," he said, tears filling his eyes. "You were not supposed to go through anything like that."

I felt his sincerity—his brotherly love.

I love you too, Cody.

* * *

My treatment team was adamant about the potential impact of substance use. Aside from probation, I had struggled with addiction in the past.

I was honest about wanting to drink, especially after the legal consequences ended.

"But I am a lot more weary of weed," I said. "I know that had a greater impact."

"When you can drink again, moderation is key," my substance use counselor said. "But try not to use it when coping with a mental health challenge."

Drugs, particularly weed based on my history, were best to avoid.

"Marijuana's psychoactive ingredient could inflame your symptoms," she said. "I wouldn't risk it."

She was right. One time, I took a puff with a friend when immediately, the world felt heavy and sporadic—lines of light snagging my attention.

I can never smoke weed again.

I smoked cigarettes to help. I loved the motion of hand to mouth and the deep exhale. I loved smoking with those in group therapy, standing outside CASA chatting about our shitty minimum wage jobs.

They complained about therapy; I'd say otherwise.

I love therapy.

Most were there for DUIs or minimal offenses. I was there because I almost killed my dad. But they didn't know unless they looked me up online, and I felt relieved to be anonymous.

I was vocal about my substance use challenges in group therapy. One day, I stood tall and drew a diagram on the whiteboard.

"I call this The Will to Say No," I said, writing out my three-step process (Table 1).

Step 1:

Consciously think of the "In the Moment Decision"...

- When a substance presents itself, take a step back and actively think about what is happening.
- Consider the substance intently and understand your ability to say yes or no.

Step 2:

Use techniques during the decision-making moment. Think about...

- ...the pros and cons of using the substance.
- ...how substance usage has impacted you and those you're connected with.

Step 3:

Find the will to say no. If you have been in therapy or jail for substance use, it is...

- ...more likely the cons outweigh the pros.
- ...more likely you and those you're connected with have been negatively impacted.

Table 1

"Coming for your check," a group member told the counselor. We all laughed. I took his comment home with me.

Maybe a career path?

* * *

My dad and I would get together often while I lived at my mom's. He took me out to dinners and local events. In October, we continued our haunted house tradition, driving two hours to Buffalo's Frightworld because we knew they were good.

I hadn't been to a haunted house since before psychosis. Although my dad and I were never scared, this one hit differently. In the Eerie State Asylum attraction, people in bloody hospital gowns ran around with knives.

"I'm gonna kill you," they screamed. "I'm gonna kill you!"

My dad and I were mature enough to look past the absurd depiction.

"Not sure how I feel about that one," he said.

"I agree—very stigmatizing."

We had talked about my mental health long before the haunted house. However, not much about the incident. It felt easier to accept things as they were.

I was in treatment. I was working. I was doing everything I had to.

My substance use counselor encouraged me to write a letter to him that addressed the incident.

"You've seen me go from a successful athlete and college student with a promising future to a criminal in jail. I know you fear another psychotic episode, and I understand. It scared me too. I don't want you to fear me. I want a good relationship with you like before.

When the incident occurred, I felt awful. The moment you left the house, I felt a rush of guilt. I was so confused and lost. I wasn't sure what was real or not. When I returned to my normal state in jail, I couldn't believe what I had done.

I am so sorry I caused so much pain. I am sorry for letting you down."

After he read the letter, he gave me a big hug.

"I really appreciated that, bud. You know I'll always be here for you."

He put his arm on my back, and I felt his trust. The more I put myself in vulnerable situations where others were supportive, the more I felt optimistic about myself and my relationships.

"Can I come home?" I asked my dad one day.

"Yes, you can," he said.

* * *

My dad's house had changed. He finished remodeling—updated floors and walls in the bedroom and dining area. Although the kitchen and living room looked the same, they didn't feel the same.

Memories created a chilling aura—a ghost-like atmosphere that rattled my insides.

Did I really attack my dad? Did I really think I was destined to save the world? How can he forgive me?

I imagined a crime scene with blood staining the floor and counters. I saw no traces, however, and I didn't want to. But part of me wished for proof it happened—uncertainty continued to be challenging to cope with.

I had a lucid nightmare on one of my first nights at home. I was aware of my slumber but couldn't move. I then heard voices of children playing outside and saw a spider crawling on the wall.

Am I alive? Am I dead?

A dark presence lingered—the feeling of a demon-like spirit watching me. I tried ignoring it, but it moved closer until it jumped on me and slashed my throat. A phantom pain pierced my neck until I woke up in the middle of the night, sweating and shaking.

I stumbled into the kitchen for water and looked at my dad's bedroom to see a newly installed lock on his door. For a while, I'd check, wondering when he could fully trust me again. For a while, I had lucid nightmares.

Other indications of my dad's need for reassurance included no knives in the home and a mental health clinic's phone number magnetized on the fridge.

When I brought up a philosophical idea once, we had to talk it out.

"What do you think, Dad? Isn't Heaven on earth? Isn't God and other creations of existence just ideas while the pursuit of happiness is what we create?"

His eyes widened.

"You're doing what you did before," he said in panic.

"I'm sorry, Dad," I said calmly. "It's not the same. I'm just working through some hard thoughts."

"How is it different this time?"

"Because I'm putting my mental health first and discussing them in therapy too."

"Okay. I just worry," he said, relaxing his voice. "Will you tell me if anything becomes worse?"

"Of course, I will. I promise."

We didn't stop having challenges. But since we continued our conversations with mental health, we continued regaining trust.

* * *

As I made progress, I could plan my return to college. I still had a degree to finish.

SUNY Geneseo expelled me when I went to jail, and I had to testify in front of a council before returning. I needed witnesses to testify on my behalf. My parents agreed.

It was a warm summer day—my first time on campus since before the incident. My parents and I entered a room where multiple people in black suits sat on one side of a long wooden table. Several mics were before us, and the design felt corporate—cold and distant.

I was by myself at the start.

"Can you tell me about the events on that day?" someone asked.

"I was extremely delusional," I said. "I never wanted to hurt my dad."

"What led to the incident, and why do you want to come back to college?" another asked.

"Ever since I quit running, I went downhill. I coped by partying and became increasingly unwell. But I'm healthy now and need my degree to move forward."

It was hard to tell if they were satisfied or not. Then they brought in my parents.

"Can you define your son's character?" they asked my dad.

"Cohen has always been kind and generous," he said. "I know he loves this school and can succeed."

"Can you talk about the events that transpired in April?"

"I don't believe he wanted to hurt me. He was unwell."

My dad struggled to keep it together—his voice cracked, and he kept his eyes down.

I looked at him—only him—and teared up.

"Cohen is doing much better now and deserves to graduate."

Thank you, Dad.

My eyes returned to those in black as they concluded the meeting. I was livid.

Where's the empathy? Would they do this for other illnesses?

Several days after testifying, I received a letter from them. Thanks to my family, I was allowed back in. Graduating felt possible again.

* * *

Throughout the year, I attended classes and completed assignments. I had passing grades in French and Humanities. Every day, graduating felt more probable. I had to think about what was next.

I felt uncertain about starting a professional career—the news articles and recent criminal record crushed my confidence. So, I thought about graduate school.

I was interested in mental health and substance use counseling. The social work field snagged my attention. However, every application asked if I was ever expelled from college.

If I don't get accepted, what am I gonna do?

I applied to three universities, and each requested info about my past. I had to accurately describe my story in less than eight hundred words—something the news wasn't capable of.

I wrote about my illness, treatment, and college success. I wrote about how my experience fueled my desire to give back—to help others with their struggles.

"In therapy, I learned how possible it is for those facing mental illness to recover and live stable, healthy lives," I said. "But we need more protective factors such as therapists, and I want to be part of that."

My parents were on board. Although I had to move hundreds of miles away and put myself in more debt, I had a clear goal and the mindset to achieve it.

The first letter arrived from Stony Brook University on Long Island, New York. My dad watched me tear open the envelope, excited and nervous. Each unfolding of the letter tightened our stomachs.

Please, let me in. Please.

"Congratulations!" the letter said. "I am delighted to inform you that you have been admitted."

My dad and I brightened with joy.

"I knew you could do it," he said, giving me another giant squeeze of relief.

I didn't wait for any other college to get back to me. I made my decision.

I'm moving forward.

* * *

By the end of spring 2017—more than one year after jail—I graduated with my bachelor's degree. Probation and conditional discharge expired. I completed the substance use program and the requirements for therapy. I was accepted into graduate school.

What else could I ask for?

I was able to decrease the dosage till I was off medication. But that didn't mean I would never take them again. I'd keep that door open—every form of treatment had to be a part of my self-management toolbox.

Graduate school was around the corner, and I had come far from my experience with mental illness. Professionally, socially, and mentally—I made leaps and bounds in my life that had once felt very uncertain.

I did everything I had to.

Persevering grit.

* * *

I thoroughly engaged in recovery. I don't think anyone can be perfect—I made mistakes smoking weed and drinking on probation. However, I invested extensive effort into support and treatment. I didn't want to waste any opportunity to improve.

Recovery is work. Recovery can be tough. Recovery is possible and even probable in the right circumstances. Mental health organizations teach the four pillars of recovery—health, home, purpose, and community—and I agree with them. I had all four.

I was in treatment for my health. My mom and dad gave me a home—a space of comfort and nourishment. I found purpose in graduating college and pursuing a career of interest. My community was accessible with work and social support—I could feel independent and connect with others facing challenges.

What if I had none of that?

People often don't live in circumstances with all four pillars, and I'm humbled to have been privileged with them. I'm terrified to think of where I would be without these supports.

Imagine someone with moderate symptoms of a mental health diagnosis—medication lowers its severity. They have their own apartment, but it's rundown and can't afford another place because of difficulty meeting basic bills. They struggle to hold a job, and disability doesn't pay enough. Forget about quality food, a space for healthy hobbies, or luxuries of any kind.

Maybe they tried to go to community college once but felt judged by others. So, in fear of connecting with people, they isolate themselves, constantly feeling sad and angry.

The family tries to help, buying groceries and saying words of encouragement. But they end up frustrated when nothing changes. This person has accepted a livelihood of poverty and unwellness.

What are the chances they can improve their life? Can we even consider them in recovery? How can anyone help when many don't have the four pillars necessary for recovery?

Do you have someone like this in your life?

What if my family didn't let me back into their lives, or I was never released from jail? What if my symptoms worsened, and I struggled to finish my degree or complete treatment? What if I wasn't accepted into graduate school—would I have felt confident moving forward with my life?

Regarding the news articles and people's ruthless comments about me, I never blamed them for demonizing me. Although it still hurts, I see their judgments as a reflection of society's misunderstanding. Violence associated with untreated mental illness is unfortunate and scary.

I get it.

But what if the response to my crisis and its recovery was similar to surviving cancer? What difference could have that made for me?

My father faced great difficulty when the incident occurred and didn't back down. His unconditional love overcame tragedy. His strength was something I remembered when the next two years brought challenges I couldn't foresee.

The first year of my recovery was just the beginning.

MIND-BODY MAINTENANCE

The color red was everywhere. From people's clothes to cement walls and plastic seats, red showed unity—or conformity, depending on how I looked at it. The stadium's immense size kept my eyes and mind busy.

I was at a basketball game in my first semester at Stony Brook University. Whistles filled the air. Trumpets and drums blared from the arena's corner. Hundreds of people chanted, "Go Seawolves! Go Seawolves!"

I felt my body dissolve—as if its entity separated and floated. From there, I sailed the sea of people, observing their movements ranging in intensity.

Each person had a role. Those in black and white stripes scanned their eyes like cameras. They danced with the players who, in matching red and white, pursued a spherical ball. Everyone else observed, cheering or booing when the moment said so.

After seeing as much as I could, I listened. Voices from every direction penetrated my mind. Adults, teenagers, and children—a mixture of souls.

Some were loud. Some were quiet. Some I could hear from afar, while some were right next to me.

Organized chaos.

I was overwhelmed at some point—uncertain if the voices were from someone's mouth or my mind. I was reminded of jail when I heard the gremlins speaking to me. At the second of this memory, an explicit statement snagged my attention.

"I bet she's pretty tight," the voice said.

I was looking at a woman in front of me. The voice paired with her and in came intrusive sexual thoughts.

What the hell?

I didn't want to think about what my mind was telling me. I didn't want to hear what I heard. I felt trapped. Subtle symptoms captured my thoughts and feelings, and I was uncomfortable.

What am I to do?

I had to handle it. I had to respond appropriately. I had to manage the overstimulation.

*Hmmm...haaa...*I took a silent pause within.

I closed my eyes. I focused on my breath. I gripped my seat.

The plastic underneath me squished like a pillow. My breath's rhythm smoothed. After a few minutes, I felt calm and grounded. I returned to my body and separated my thoughts from the potential psychosis symptoms.

It's just a basketball game. It's just a basketball game.

I saw nothing extraordinary about the basketball game.

* * *

Te te te te te te te te. Din din din din din din din din. Loud noises repeated.

I sought rhythm—a pattern to comfort me—but couldn't. So, as instructed, I focused on the tiny white dot centering the computer's black display. Like the round bolt fixed to the jail cell wall, I found relief in a motionless, circular speck.

I was participating in a psychiatric study at Yale University. Although it reminded me of my mind's captivity, I felt privileged to contribute to mental illness research.

An hour into the CT scan, I felt uneasy. I wasn't bored—my thoughts kept me busy. But pain formed at my skull's base. If only I could've shifted positions or drank water.

"Alright Cohen, we're starting again," a researcher said.

The computer screen flashed on. The tiny white dot returned, and I readied, gripping a joystick with a finger over a button.

"Don't forget. Do not move your head."

With focus, my eyes did not leave the dot.

Te te te te te te te te. Din din din din din din din din. The machine turned back on.

A yellow circle appeared and disappeared on the screen. I, using the joystick, moved a white circle to where it existed. Seeing a straight line to its exact spot, I wanted to match it perfectly—determined as the challenge happened over and over.

Eyes steady—the white dot turned blue, and I pushed the button before it changed back.

I never miss that cue.

Another hour passed. Then another. I repeated the tasks, so my mind would activate how the researchers wanted it to.

At one point, I imagined eternal beings disguised themselves as the researchers. I'd see them through the bottom slits of my eyes, wearing black headphones. They studied my brain—*my brain*—because of its discovery.

Maybe I'm the next human to join their eternity.

I was prepped for the scan. When getting ready, someone resembled a man in black from jail.

"I'm uncomfortable," I told a researcher. "Like I'm back in jail…that man was there."

"He's a lab technician," she said. "Let me introduce him to you."

The researcher then described the black headphones and stillness. It became easier to manage potential symptoms. Especially bizarre thoughts of eternal beings studying my mind.

Is that happening or probable? No. Is it possible? Sure.

Absurdity was just that—an endless list of possibilities to imagine. However, I realized how bizarre my thoughts were.

I don't believe eternal beings are studying me. I don't believe my brain is extraordinary.

I shifted my perspective, viewing these thoughts as an imagination akin to sci-fi.

Like *The Matrix.*

* * *

On many occasions throughout graduate school, the connection between my mind, body, and reality dissolved.

Sometimes beautiful. Sometimes troubling.

Always something to be aware of.

When I didn't feel like Cohen or what society expected of me—like conforming to a basketball spectator or feeling extraterrestrial—symptoms like intrusive and bizarre thoughts were revealed. I'd make a note and inform my college therapist who helped me navigate these experiences.

He connected my out-of-mind-and-body encounters with derealization, a feeling that what surrounds you doesn't exist, and depersonalization, a feeling of not existing. An insight that mirrored my feelings and allowed me to understand better.

I must continue learning how to manage my health.

The stigma I continued to face didn't help. A campus office hired me as a student assistant, and within the first few weeks, I sensed rejection.

"I don't want you to be overwhelmed..." Joan, my supervisor said. "Not with schizophrenia."

They must've found those news articles.

Even in my social work program, presumptions were made behind my back.

"I'm worried about having Cohen in class," a student told a new friend of mine.

I'm not a bad person, though.

I was caring for my health. I was making progress.

Do I not deserve to be here?

* * *

In the second semester of my first year, symptoms challenged me even more. On an early morning, I was in the library's quiet section—a perfect place for silent thoughts and space to work on a large white desk.

I have to work with paper.

Ink stained my fingers. Eraser clumps sprinkled my shirt. Books piled a few inches high.

Each paper I worked on had a reason. Graphs, numbers, and letters—squiggles only I knew the meaning of. I switched between pen and pencil—one for certainty while the other gave room for mistakes.

"If we, in mind-and-body, spend our limited time..." I wrote. "...we can teach ourselves and each other to want love in all that exists through God."

I knew I didn't believe in God when I wrote the paragraph. I tried to be as objective as I could.

So, what did I mean by God?

I eventually figured it out. God was an acronym for the Generation of Organized Dimensions. It meant anything I could perceive or experience would have to be generated into a thing of being through dimensional organization.

They're the words to describe how things come into reality—the source of all things.

My conclusion filled me with a desire to search more—to know more. But the hours spent in the library weren't enough. My campus job started soon.

I left to inform Joan of my needed absence. But something felt off.

My body was coordinated with the environment—a floating sensation. Colors pulsated with gracious shades. Campus signs designed to inspire students caught my eye like they were meant to.

Although partly beautiful, I worried that I could lose control. I then saw an older man with white hair and a silver mustache. He resembled someone I felt strangely attached to.

$e = mc2$

I had been examining Einstein's equation that morning. The man appeared at the precise time and location.

An eerie connection infiltrated my mind. Fear thumped my chest and stomach.

I wondered what was actually happening.

Something seems wrong.

My slight questioning made me think differently—respond differently. I was able to get off work. Instead of returning to the library, I chose to eat lunch. I wasn't hungry but told myself I needed food.

The dining hall was busy and loud. So many people doing things and going places. I wanted to tune everything out.

I put on my black noise-canceling headphones. I kept them with me for stressful situations. I turned on a soft instrumental playlist and sat at a booth to eat.

In less than a few minutes, the man who resembled Einstein appeared at a table near me.

Ding ding ding. A noise I had never heard before rang from my smartphone.

Huh?

I always turned off sound notifications on my smartphone. When I looked, my fear doubled.

An app I never used prompted the news article "Stephen Hawking Dies on Einstein's Birthday."

I looked at the date—March 14, 2018—and remembered it was my mom's birthday.

Did Einstein and I have a connection I'm not aware of?

My bones shuddered with paranoia—skin slipping off my skeleton.

Is the universe sending me a message? Am I here—alive in this booth?

I was lost in thought for several minutes. When I looked at the man, he had disappeared.

Did I hallucinate him?

Panic bubbled my throat. My heart throbbed with alarm. I was more than out of mind and body. I was drowning.

I wanted it to stop. I wanted to feel okay. Then it clicked.

I was unwell.

Very unwell.

I immediately closed my eyes and composed myself. I gripped my hands together and focused on the piano and strings.

Whiiisss... whooosss... whiiisss... whooosss... whiiisss... whooosss. I could feel the sound of breath through my nostrils.

After a few minutes, I opened my eyes.

I need to take care of myself.

Now.

* * *

I left the dining hall and found a bench. For a long while, I sat, listening to the birds.

The day was sunny. The air was cool. As the sun rounded my head, a few hours passed, and the world felt calmer—I felt rested. When the time was right, I analyzed what happened.

I thought about my work. Each week, I spent twenty hours at my campus job, ten hours in class, fourteen hours of field placement, and constant school work. On top of responsibilities, I embraced a philosophy that sometimes became a priority.

Why am I doing so much?

I knew why I pursued philosophy. I struggled to avoid existential thoughts.

Does reality come from within the mind or the other way around? If my brain holds the gift of life, and it's not found beyond the skies, where does it begin? Where does it end?

I didn't lose sight of how philosophy influenced my mental health. But I couldn't ignore it either. To cope, I'd recall the waterless desert illustrated by Albert Camus in *The Myth of Sisyphus.*

In Greek mythology, Sisyphus taught us to accept our failures as we do our achievements. Camus approached existential thought similarly, exploring the mind in ways a CT scan could never. For me, his waterless desert represented a path in which thought, being pushed to its furthest boundaries, could discover its confines.

Maybe I have no life when searching for the answers to life.

I didn't stop there though. I spoke honestly to my therapist.

"Proceed with caution," he'd say.

He didn't think I should avoid philosophy. I just couldn't allow myself to be consumed by it. The way I saw it, anytime I'd enter the labyrinth of philosophical thought, I'd have to keep a string wrapped around me, ready to pull me out if psychosis intervened.

Mental illness can linger. Mental illness can wax and wane. Mental illness can return with cunning force.

I had to realize that.

I have to realize that.

* * *

At some point, I connected with my professor of Social Policy and Social Determinants. His bio listed spirituality as an interest of study.

"How does spirituality relate to social work?" I asked.

"A lot of people have difficulty finding meaning," he said. "A social worker can help with that."

Makes sense.

"What do you think of this sentence? 'Eternal life is the balance of thinking and doing while feeling both.'"

I had changed "occurs when you balance" to "is the balance of" because it felt more logical.

We don't know if one can obtain eternal life. But assuming humans are the same as me, our reality's entirety is experienced through the balance—even if we're not always perceiving the balance.

"That's very Zen," he said.

He recommended Robert Pirsig's *Zen and the Art of Motorcycle Maintenance*. The story about a journey with philosophy—sometimes beautiful, sometimes troubling—made me feel I wasn't alone.

I had never read philosophical fiction before, but it quickly became a favorite. The next time I saw the professor, I asked if we could meet about it. He agreed.

I was in a healthy state of mind in our meeting.

"I sometimes struggle to understand how I exist...how you exist," I said. "Isn't it possible for anything outside my immediate perception to not be there?"

"Anything is possible," he said. "It's possible for a jet engine to land on us right now. But it's highly unlikely, right? That's the challenge with disregarding the scientific method."

Interesting...probabilities matter.

We would meet a half-dozen times—always analyzing philosophers, music, and art. He gave me more books. *Siddhartha* by Hermann Hesse, *The Alchemist* by Paulo Coelho, and *John Livingston Seagull* by Richard Bach. I found a new appreciation for Greek mythology and museums like the Metropolitan Museum of Art.

I never had a philosophical role model before—someone who engaged in meaningful conversation no matter how abstract or absurd. For so long I dealt with challenging ideas on my own. But now, I felt heard.

The professor conveyed the need for attention to self and wellness, expressing the importance of remaining grounded and respecting the ideas of others.

"Remember, that is what you see," he'd say. "That is your idea."

He was right: my view was my belief. If my belief helped me grasp reason and reality, it served its purpose. It may not be the same as others, and that's okay.

That is okay.

I understood.

A beautiful simplicity among complex uncertainty.

* * *

Although graduate school challenged my mental health, it supported me too. Throughout the two years, I developed a healthy routine. I quit cigarettes. I enjoyed running again. After years of not lacing up, I finally saw it as a way to maintain wellness—not a necessity for success.

I was as social as I needed to be, staying connected to loved ones and making new friends. For the most part, I drank in moderation. But some nights were a struggle.

I once fell into a garbage bag on Manhattan streets because I was so drunk. Another time I burst out in tears—one of the many times I cried about my past. These nights served as more reminders of my need to care for mental health.

I worked hard at my campus job and in school. I took initiative, executing a project that I received a grant for. I organized and led events, collaborating well with university staff and students.

I was nominated for Student Employee of the Year. I was accepted into the Phi Alpha Honor Society for my 3.94 GPA and extensive community service.

My future felt promising.

What's next?

* * *

I received full support when applying for jobs. Everyone was willing to write a recommendation letter—quite a different tone from my first few weeks.

Somebody at the university told me the news articles were discovered soon after I arrived. Many people felt alarmed. But once they learned who I was and the work I could do, concerns about my past disappeared.

That didn't stop the articles from haunting me, however.

"Google yourself," the career center would say. "See what employers might see."

Who would want to hire me?

I contacted the five news stations, hoping they'd remove the articles.

"I am telling you this because I've never wanted to hurt anyone," I emailed. "As I pursue a social work career, employers will likely search my name. I don't want this article to be their first impression of me and jeopardize my career."

Three didn't reply. Two responded with doubt.

"Are there any factual errors in the article?" a staff member said. "We can only remove an article if there are factual errors."

What assholes.

I attended a presentation by someone with lived experience of mental illness.

"What can I do about these news articles?" I asked the presenter.

"Ignore them. Let them go and focus on you," she said.

That stuck with me. Soon after, I wrote an article for the National Alliance on Mental Illness.

"I've realized that hiding the stigma I experienced from those articles wouldn't help prevent it for myself or others," I wrote. "Instead, I'm writing as a self-advocate, using my voice to help change the perception of mental illness."

Maybe employers will see that first.

* * *

My studies were personally and professionally beneficial. I learned how social issues were reflected in the individual, community, and society. I improved my communication and saw the importance of empathy. I learned about mental health and treatment from a clinical perspective.

Instead of direct service, I pursued the macro route of social work—community, policy, and political social action.

We need systemic and cultural changes in mental health.

I remembered when I first went to the hospital, no one gave me cards like they do for physical illness. So, for a school project, I created Hopeful Notes—cards similar to get-well cards but designed for supporting a loved one in a mental health crisis.

I met with peers at a local mental health clinic. After sharing a bit about my mental illness, I read a hopeful note.

"Your beautiful mind makes you one of a kind. As you conquer any challenges you find, I'll be there, loving you all time."

We worked together on more poems for the concept.

"Thank you for doing this," a peer said.

I found myself in a unique position to give back—to help others.

This is my destiny.

* * *

When graduation neared, I was ready to walk across that stage. I was ready to move on with my life. However, I had yet to find a job—to find future certainty.

How?

I felt so much inspiration from my family, friends, and colleagues on graduation day. But as soon as I returned home, hope diminished as quickly as my mental health did.

My journey wasn't over—*it never would be.* The next challenge to my mental health brought me to a similar point when I had to go to the hospital.

A crisis was upon me once again.

Could I survive it?

Enduring pressure.

* * *

My college therapist diagnosed me with mildly severe schizoaffective disorder. It includes schizophrenia symptoms like delusions and bipolar symptoms like mania. Mild severity means symptoms have an infrequent presence and impact.

I never felt the need for a diagnosis—still don't. Although they can help us understand mental health, sometimes, I feel they can add barriers too.

People might focus on the diagnosis, not the person. People might feel like it's an all-or-nothing situation, such as blaming illness for every behavior or not acknowledging how people vary.

The term disorder also makes it feel like mental illness is a defect, which I know is not the case. I've gained a lot of hope and insight by managing my mental health, particularly among psychosis.

So no, I don't see myself having a disorder. Rather, I see it as a diagnosis. One that doesn't hurt to know because I care more about managing my specific experiences instead of the label. One that gives me knowledge to better support my mental health and a recognition of my responsibility in taking care of myself.

Which I did.

I managed typical stressors such as balancing the hats of a student, office worker, and intern. I managed the symptoms I still faced. When overwhelmed, however, symptoms severity increased, and I had to act more urgently.

I was slipping into a potentially critical situation when I believed I saw Einstein whose birthday was that day. Was he a hallucination or a member of the campus? I don't know. Was the notification spurred by delusion or absurd coincidence? I don't know.

Sometimes, weird shit just happens without explanation, and I've had to come to terms with that. No matter what, I had to take care of myself immediately, and I'm glad I did.

What if I didn't realize how unwell I was in the dining hall—would I have been in crisis? What if I didn't have someone like the professor—someone who helped me cope with existential dread? What if my difficulties in graduate school prevented me from graduating?

I had come so far, obtaining a master's degree within three years of jail. I am so appreciative of everything that brought me to this point, including my hard work. However, I still faced major obstacles.

Getting a job was more challenging than I thought it would be. I quickly learned that continuing to manage my mental health would be even more difficult.

BACK ON TRACK

Driving home alone, I had to squint my eyes to seek comfort in the hills. It was late afternoon, and the sun hovered below my car's sun visor. Scattered clouds decorated the distant trees with rose-colored embers.

I was returning from an interview at Stony Brook University—a job I desperately wanted. However, Joan, who was on the hiring committee, hinted that it didn't go well.

"You brought a lot of energy," she said. "Keep looking. I'm here to help if you need it."

I was used to being shut down from jobs. I failed more than ten interviews before and after graduating. But for some reason, my mind was on fire after this one.

Over and over on the seven-hour drive, I analyzed every exchange I could recall. Memories of other unsuccessful interviews crept in—times when I rambled too fast and long. Sometimes, I wasn't thinking of interviews but previous mistakes.

Maybe it's my past.

Part of me felt I wouldn't get the job because of mania—the upbeat, bouncing from one idea to the next, I had to say everything symptom. The pathways of my neurons had been burning, and their cracks were showing.

I couldn't keep my mouth shut and listen.

Embarrassing. How do I keep failing?

My struggle to cope worsened. Stress-induced and fear-driven thoughts gripped the steering wheel. I—*my brain*—was a ticking time bomb.

For a moment, I considered buying a bottle of booze. I knew it wouldn't help, but at least its depressant effect would slow down my mind. However, I made it home before the temptation hijacked the best of me.

* * *

The sky was dark by the time I stepped through the front doors.

"How'd the interview go?" my dad asked with a pep in his step.

"I think it went well," I said. "We can hope."

That's all I ever do is hope.

But it was a lie—my bullshit optimism. I didn't want my dad to know, and I wasn't feeling vulnerable.

In my bedroom, the physical silence of the night wasn't enough to quiet the loudness in my head. Thought after thought.

I must've talked too much. She didn't get to ask a question. I should've stopped talking.

Question after question.

Why did I pull my phone out? Why were their faces red? Did I discuss how I discovered that huge indicator of success in my data report?

Pulse after pulse. It felt like a tidal wave was brewing in the pit of my skull, and I was letting it swell. I couldn't lie still.

As my body shifted and flipped, desperately trying to rest, running medals behind my bed clanked and clattered. Other walls of my childhood room displayed plaques and trophies—pictures of friends and posters of concerts. They were all memories of a life

I grew out of. For then, I lie with a life that—for some reason—I couldn't grow into.

I glanced at my clock to see it was four in the morning.

Why can't I sleep?

Paranoia soon seeped from the dark corners of my room—a place of solace. Sporadic thoughts—some intrusive, some abstract—infiltrated my nerves. When I questioned recent events, my mind latched onto improbable answers.

Maybe my old therapist was at the store because they knew I was unwell. Maybe I didn't get the job because they saw me as evil. Maybe I should've worn a different colored suit.

I felt my thoughts steering my perception into an obscured horizon. Then my neighbor's porch light—a single dot beaming sharp lines of light into my room—looked a bit too symmetrical.

This isn't good.

An alarm of serious unwellness began to ring. Something told me I needed help. Immediate help. But what was I to do when mania-induced psychosis struck its match at four in the morning?

I considered waking up my dad to go to the hospital. I considered calling Finn. However, I feared them panicking or becoming afraid of me.

I'll wait till the morning.

* * *

As I chose to handle the situation independently, I did what I knew I could do. I put on my black headphones—over-the-ear and noise-canceling. I turned on a meditation soundtrack. I closed my eyes and focused on the sounds of nature.

I held my hands together at my chest. I felt my breath move up and down. I repeated a favorite mantra.

I am here. I am home.

Again and again, I breathed and said the mantra. Bit by bit, I felt some form of control. Bit by bit, I felt my thoughts ease, and the fire in my mind dwindle.

Rest is coming.

In a sudden flash, it was six in the morning. Daylight shone through the window, and I made it through the night with two hours of sleep. I wanted to sleep more, but I felt jittery and restless. So I moved through the kitchen and to the living room.

There I sat, in the same room where my dad and I slow-danced when I was little. The same room where we watched TV and talked about my future. The same room where the blade tip nearly punctured his throat.

I patiently waited for him to wake up, so I could tell him what was happening. He eventually stumbled out of his bedroom, plopped in his recliner, and grabbed the remote—as he had done for many years. But before he turned on the TV, I spoke.

"Dad, I'm not feeling well," I said.

"Like a cold or something?" he asked.

"No, mentally. I feel off and not myself."

He sat up and made eye contact with me.

"I know it's been stressful for you getting a job, and I have sensed something has been off. What's going on?"

I told him about my racing thoughts, lack of sleep, and how I was very aware of my state.

"I don't want you to panic," I added. "But I need help right now."

"Okay, what can we do?"

I suggested the hospital. But since the space felt safe, I considered other treatment ideas. The emergency room was the last resort.

My dad researched local resources. He found a nearby mental health clinic that allowed for crisis intervention therapy, similar to urgent care for physical illness. I could start there before deciding on the hospital.

He called them, and I had an appointment within a few hours.

Thank you, Dad.

* * *

My dad dropped me off at the clinic. I walked in, nervous and eager—my feet balancing on a tightrope.

Am I going to be okay?

I clamped my hands while the secretary gave me a form and clipboard. I firmly held a pen, slowly scanning each word, so I could interpret every question accurately. After returning the form, I sat in the corner and closed my eyes until someone called my name.

"Is Cohen here?" a man asked.

I took a deep breath and stood.

"I'm here."

He directed me to his office. As I walked in, I immediately felt warm and tranquil. Soft yellow lamps illuminated the space. Small fountains trickled water down their curved stone.

A framed quote on the wall said, "Within you, there is a stillness and a sanctuary to which you can retreat at any time and be yourself."

Is this office designed for someone with mania?

I loved it.

"What brings you here?" the therapist asked.

"I feel like I am about to have a psychotic break," I said. "I've considered going to the hospital."

I described my mental health diagnosis and history of mental illness. I told him about graduate school and my inability to get a job. I explained the day and night before, and how I was very willing to do whatever it took to get help, including going back on meds.

He listened. He asked questions. He thanked me for coming to him.

"You'd have to meet with our psychiatrist to get prescribed, and we can consider that in the near future," he said. "But for now, let's focus on you getting rested."

He suggested for the next several days, I concentrate on the most basic duties of day-to-day life. This included showering, eating, sleeping, and doing chores.

"What about running?" I asked.

"If you feel like you can go for a run, go for a run. But it may not be the best idea if stress is associated with it."

We talked about music.

"I've had a history of seeing signs," I said. "But I think instrumental music is okay because there are no words. Plus, it's always helped me relax."

"If that works for you, I'm all for it," he said.

By the end of our session, I had already felt better. It turns out I didn't have to go to the hospital. I had to relax. I had to take a break from pursuing jobs.

I had to focus on my health.

* * *

I saw the therapist each week for the remainder of the summer. I didn't have to take medication because I managed my symptoms. When the time felt right, I applied for jobs. With the help of my therapist, family, and friends—*my support network*—I approached my interviews differently.

Instead of compiling a list of ideas to share with interviewers and trying to remember everything, I focused on my presence in the room. Where were my hands? What was my posture like? What could I do to feel more comfortable and grounded in the space?

Joan suggested holding my hands together when not talking. I recalled how that helped me ground myself when symptomatic.

I remembered the importance of breathing.

Hooo…ahhh…hooo…haaa…hooo…haaa…

I stepped back. I embraced patience. I practiced interviewing with my new intention.

The more I practiced, the more I felt determination and courage—qualities I learned as a runner—give me the strength to carry on. It wasn't long before I had another interview.

The job's title was Project Coordinator. With the Mental Health Association in New York State, I would work on the School Mental Health Resource and Training Center—a project supporting a recent policy requiring NYS kindergarten through twelfth grade schools to provide mental health instruction in health classes.

I was impressed that my state was the first to pass a law requiring mental health education in schools.

Could have that made a difference for me?

At the first interview, I made my adjustments. I took deep breaths. I gripped my hands when not talking. I trusted myself—and it worked. They called me back for the second round.

In September 2019, I was hired. I finally felt a sense of security and hope again. I could finally feel comfortable with my future.

I made it.

Not only did I make it, but I found myself in a position that could alleviate the suffering of others, prevent tragedies, and enact real change.

I never forgot how significantly different my life would have been if I killed my dad. I never forgot how the incident could've been prevented. I never forgot how my dad and I had to rely on a miracle to save our lives.

What's next?

* * *

Although the incident had been three years prior—three years of hard work to secure the next step in my life—I still struggled. I still had to improve upon managing my mental health. I still had to realize how mental illness can linger, wax and wane, and return with cunning force.

The night I struggled with mania, it was risky to handle it alone. If I knew about the crisis hotline, I could've called them. But shame, stigma, and lack of knowledge controlled me more than my diagnosis.

My dad, however, gave me the best support. He was patient. He actively listened to my needs. We worked together to get help.

Perhaps that was what I meant when I told Finn the incident would make him and me closer.

We could have never had that conversation before.

* * *

On a warm fall day, my dad drove me to Albany, New York—our state's capital city. We had a list of apartments to look at—my job was starting soon.

A musky-sweet smell suffused the air. Trees were just starting to change color, orange and red seeping through their green leaves.

From Interstate 86, we took the same route I'd take to Long Island until the road diverged, and we traveled north on I-88. It was a road I had yet to take but one where my journey continued.

For hours we drove through the rolling hills of upstate, rocking out to our favorite bands Breaking Benjamin and Staind. We passed attractions we visited when I was a child—the Corning Museum of Glass and the village of Watkins Glen. The road was calm, and I felt sentimental, realizing how far I had come to get where I was going.

I recalled a moment two days before the incident. I had imagined getting married and traveling the world to spread my word. In the dead of night, when leaving for the church with the big red doors, I paused to look at my home.

I remembered feeling sad, thinking I'd never live there again. Although I was delusional, missing my dad was genuine. Now that I was officially moving out, the sadness was even more real.

I looked at him in the driver's seat. His age was showing—white hair thinning, face drooping. But his eyes sparkled.

"What do you think, Dad? You'll visit in October?"

He smiled.

"Of course. Has to be a good haunted house somewhere here."

He had done so much for me. He was at every race. He gave me more than I ever needed.

I wouldn't be where I am without him.

"Can't wait," I said. "Maybe we'll finally get scared."

"Ha! Maybe," he laughed.

Thank you, Dad.

Thank you.

Even when the dark side of life reared its ugly head, he cared for me.

He loved me.

And I'll never stop loving him.

Thank you for guiding me in my journey.

Forever grateful.

Onward.

Hi Bud! I Love you. You mean everything to me. The mess you are going through is going to take some time to fix. You will need to be patient and do what doctors say. We will get you through this. The state will not allow gram and I to have any contact with you, so your mom will communicate between you and me if you want. Do you need anything. We are here to help and get you through this. I've had so many people contact to wish good luck and Love to you. We are all here to help. This may be a good moment to write your movie. Just ask for help. I miss you and am thinking of you.

Letter from Dad

Cohen, 4.21.16

Hey Brother! First I want you to know I am here for you and I think about you everyday and all your going through. As I grow older I realize more and more how tough life is and how the bond between siblings is so strong and nothing can break it. This all seems so unreal that your in this situation. I wish there was a way I could help. I pray for you mom and your Dad daily. We will all stay here and strong for you because thats what family is for, and we are blessed to have eachother..... I truly hope your given the help and tools you need to move on from all this and live that happy healthy successful life youve worked so hard for and deserve. Feel free to call (585-491-3265) or write me I am always here for you. I sent some photos you might want to keep with you to remind you how much we all love and care about you and always will. Love Karmen ♡

Letter from Karmen

Dear Cohen,

I hope you're okay. I've been
thinking about you alot. You can't imagine
that I think of you every day now.

The conditions you're in, the cold
floor, bare walls and minimal windows
it too shall pass.

When in the situation your in
It can be real comforting and
entertaining to give in to the impulses
You've gotta concentrate on whats
in front of you.

Find laughter :)

I love you babiest brother
You had one life going for you,
You can find another

Good Luck in there.
Take it in like it a new journey.

I Love you
Lindsay

Letter from Lindsay

①

Ooooh Brother! Where art thou? :P (good ass movie)
So I just got home from visiting with you.
I tell ya what That was harder than I
thought it would be. It kills me to see you
in there, you dont belong there. if I could
I would stay with you until you could leave.
but since you told me youre just super bored
I thought Id write to you - (forgot to space ha)
to pass the time. I dont really know what
to write about.. Oooo but 1 thing. I will
NEVER move to florida :P its just a
vacation spot haha... theres too many
people and you have to pay for parking
EVERYWHERE... its rediculous. the only
GREAT thing about it was the beach
and the ocean and Steak-n-Shake
I think the first order of business when you
get out is food. You wanna go to a
buffet orrrr make one at home? :P
I want you to know that you have a
HUUUUGE support system of people
waiting for you when you get home.
Everyone misses you like crazy & I
for sure can not wait to just be able
to chill and jam out or go for hikes.
→

Letter from Casie

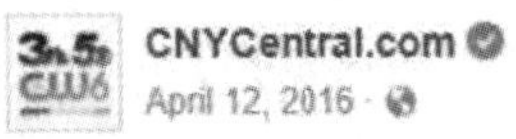

CNYCentral.com
April 12, 2016

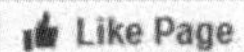

Like Page

Troopers say 22-year-old Cohen Miles-Rath attacked his father with a kitchen knife and then bit off a chunk of his earlobe when his father tried to take the knife ou: of his hands.

He was caught by troopers who saw him leaving the home with his father's blood on him.

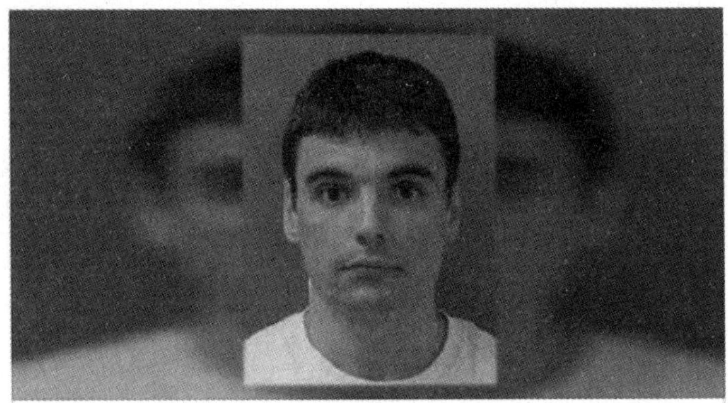

Troopers: Man bites off part of father's earlobe during fight

Cohocton, N.Y. - A Steuben County man is facing charges after State Police said he bit off a portion of his father's earlobe during a fight.Around 1 p.m. Monday,...

CNYCENTRAL.COM

The Facebook news article post

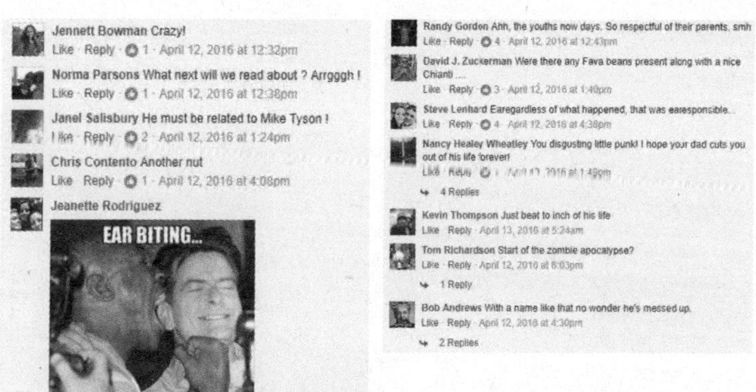

Comments on the Facebook news article post

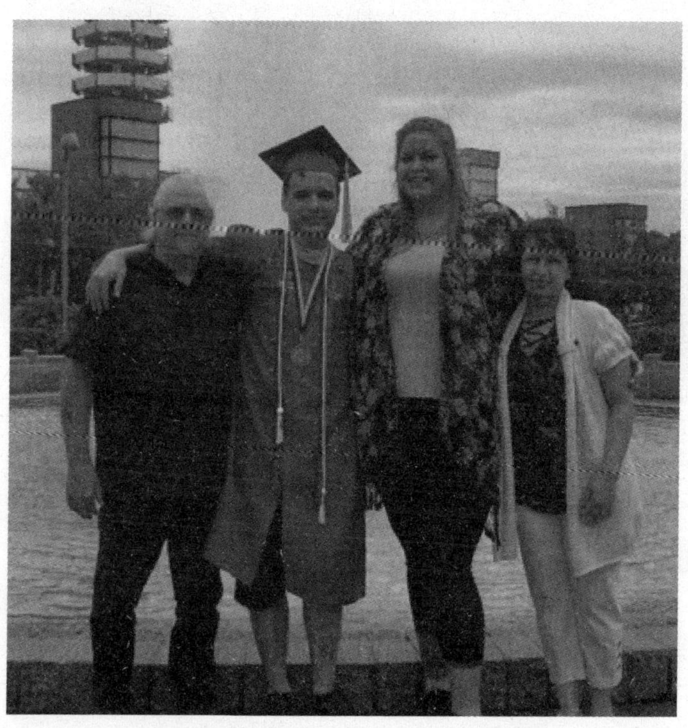

Left to right: Dad, Cohen, Casie, and Mom

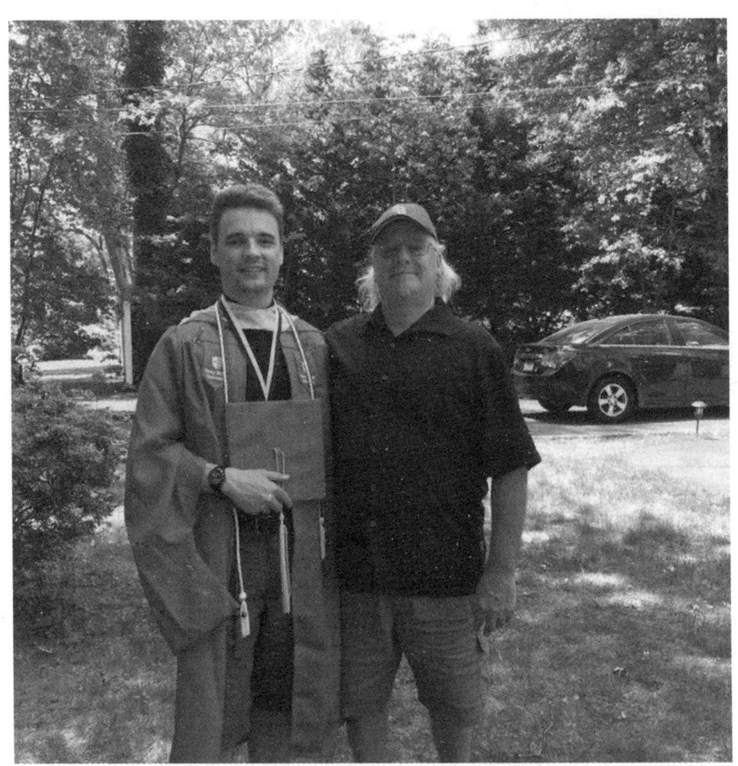

Cohen and Dad at MSW graduation

EPILOGUE

I wouldn't be where I am today if the result of my illness had been different. If I killed my father, I'd be in prison or a psychiatric hospital like Timothy Granata. Or, on the day of the incident, I could've been murdered by the police like Daniel Prude.

Yet here I am, similar to Elyn R. Saks, who survived, wrote a memoir about her experience, and seeks change through mental health law, policy, and ethics.

I was more likely to survive a mental health crisis and thrive afterward. The early intervention of my diagnosis—which only became effective after the incident—and the support and resources from my family, friends, and community guided my recovery.

Not all people have these privileges.

Guidance for recovery isn't always available. Treatment may not be accessible or effective. Families may have difficulty providing support. Communities may not treat mental health as an integral part of overall health. Therefore, recovery progress falls short, and people continue to be significantly impacted by illness.

Mental illness can also be relentless and debilitating, making it harder for someone to surmount. No matter how we perceive someone's ability to overcome, such as success in the traditional sense, every positive health change is significant and deserves to be honored.

When struggling to overcome, we must lift up, give reasons to have hope, and celebrate as the attempts are made. Just like physical illness, mental illness varies. Healing and hope look very different for every person.

Since working in the mental health field, I've recognized changes we can make to lessen the impact of mental health challenges and reduce the likelihood of mental illness causing people to suffer. Changes include but are not limited to:

- make social and emotional intelligence the goal of childhood development, fostering it in the home, academics, extracurricular activities, and beyond
- embed mental health literacy in the educational system, including its connection to whole-body health, knowledge of mental illnesses, and an understanding of risk and protective factors for wellness
- ingrain mental health support in systems of care, making support such as therapy and community-based services viable
- develop an integrated healthcare and social care system that effectively addresses social determinants of health
- expand and improve research that advances an understanding of mental health and wellness, including impact, intersectionality, and support practices
- dismantle structural barriers, such as poverty, that increase financial fragility, racial tension, and other social issues, as they can often narrow the path

individuals and communities can take to manage health and wellness

- shift jail practices from punitive to restorative to reduce recidivism—potential in saving taxpayer money—and support health and wellness
- raise the voices of peers—those with lived experience of mental illness—and the services they can provide to help people
- take action with our mental health by engaging with it regularly and shifting the culture of how we respond when faced with a challenge and/or illness
- create a space among family, friends, and communities to care for mental health as an integral part of overall health, and reduce shame and stigma

Some issues are important to debate such as medication use, the impact of marijuana and other substances on mental health, and law enforcement's role in a crisis. These issues don't have easy answers, but it's essential to recognize the many perspectives and supporting research.

Something to discuss further.

Regarding violence and mental illness, I feel it is better to focus on improving our efforts with prevention, intervention, and crisis response rather than the tragic result when support isn't achieved.

Stories like Timothy's and Daniel's can help us engage in deeper conversations about mental health. I hope my story has done that for you. If one change I listed had been made before the incident with my father, we might not have had to rely on a miracle to save our lives.

* * *

I wrote this story to make sense of my experience with mental illness. In my process, I've realized how complex that is, particularly with psychosis and its unique challenges.

I've always been influenced by the culmination of my history, views, who I am—white, straight, male—and where I was born. But the specific route of my mind during psychosis leaves me with questions.

What is the meaning of the sentence I created?

My professor in graduate school viewed it as a holistic Zen-like statement. Others have told me that, when removing "eternal life," it is connected to Cognitive Behavior Therapy—treatment to help someone manage their thoughts, feelings, and behavior. The reference to "eternal life," however, makes the statement less logical and, with the state I was in, delusional as it led me to believe I was a God.

Was the sentence my mind's way of trying to pursue wellness?

I've never strongly believed in metaphysical conclusions from religion, science, or philosophy. I'm not claiming any truth about life and existence such as with the sentence. Interpretations are beyond my responsibility. But the connection between my experience and this thought process is evident.

Being symptomatic while taking Humanities impacted my thinking. Dynamic and hierarchical religious systems (Western and Eastern religions) and methodological systems of thought and study (philosophy and science) were accessible and pertinent to me.

Existential dread then brought upon my desire to seek answers. Not just to know but to feel a sense of purpose, value, and meaning—a sense of being well.

Other cases of people with psychosis have shown an association with religion, science, and philosophy. Although it's never the same experience, the similarities are an interesting look at how psychosis can shape someone's thoughts.

A philosopher like Aristotle might have argued madness can come from a mind pushing the boundaries of thought. With Albert Camus's metaphor of the waterless desert, we can think about a journey into the desert (of thought) without water (reason) and how it can result in death by dehydration (madness).

It is within the desert—of grasping what is true and what is not—that, I think, coping with psychosis meets its greatest difficulty. When I faced severe symptoms, my existential search did more harm than good. But now, it's a journey I've been able to use to support wellness.

I do not need to determine the ultimate truth of reality. I understand the delusion psychosis forced upon me. I don't believe I am a prophet or that the sentence is special. I continue pursuing philosophy, but it is just a hobby. Like my love for distance running and storytelling, my wellness doesn't rely on it.

I can cope within the desert.

* * *

Mental health has been my priority since I began writing this memoir when hired at the Mental Health Association in New York State. I continue managing challenges and maintaining wellness. I'll never forget that my diagnosis could become severe again.

Since I've been in a position to be the advocate I've wanted to be, I have taken action. In my four years of work, I have facilitated dozens of mental health training including Mental Health First Aid and Introduction to Trauma-Sensitive Schools.

Through grassroots efforts, lobbying, and communication strategies, I have advocated for mental health policies such as increased mental health workforce funding. The workforce is highly underpaid and understaffed, especially compared to other healthcare professions.

I have intertwined my advocacy with my mental health story, publicly speaking for audiences of schools, peers, government officials, and more. I once shared my story at a mental health roundtable that included the US Department of Health and Human Services Secretary Xavier Becerra (shown on page 280). In the conversation about the Bipartisan Safer Communities Act—a law implementing changes to the mental health system, school safety programs, and gun safety laws—I made my voice heard.

Whenever others discuss violence and mental health, I want to give my input. Whenever I think of Daniel being killed or Timothy in an institution, I want to scream at the system that failed to help. Whenever someone judges another person or circumstance, particularly people with mental illness, I want them to be more empathetic.

I want my experience to reveal the changes we can make and embrace the hope that comes with it. The hope I find after the attempted murder of my father. The hope I find after lying naked on a jail floor, shrieking at the terror in my mind. The hope that has been with me since I was a child.

If my feelings of uncertainty with life, existence, and the realities of our world have taught me anything, it is that I can take charge of them. I can repair the despair. I can embrace optimism. I can embody reality's complexity, simplicity, and absurdity, and still find a way to feel okay—to be well and happy.

I never do this alone, either.

I'm always seeking knowledge and connections with people. I'm always listening to their stories and perspectives. Now, I've shared my story with the world. If it has helped me mend reality, maybe it could do the same for others.

END

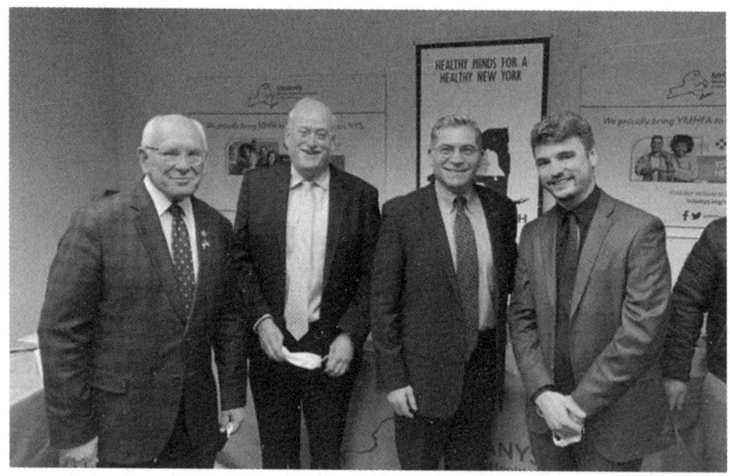

Left to right: Congressman Paul D. Tonko, Glenn Liebman (CEO of the Mental Health Association in NYS), US Secretary of Health and Human Services Xavier Becerra, and Cohen

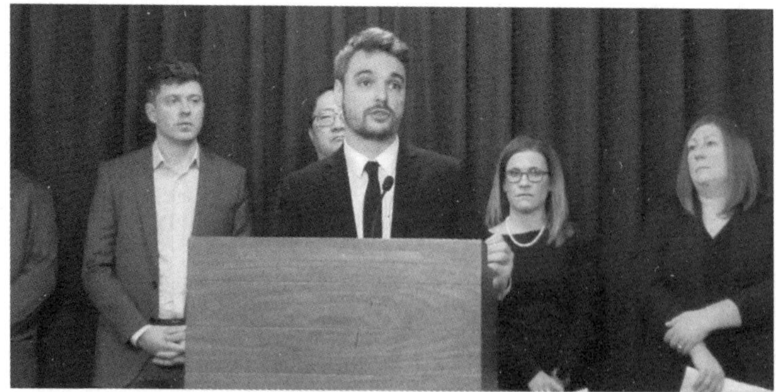

Cohen sharing story at a press conference about mental health

For those who have lost their lives to mental illness, and who currently struggle.
I see you.

For everyone who has supported me.
I am grateful.

For the advocates, and their contributions to mental health change.
I am honored to join you.

MENTAL HEALTH RESOURCES

988 Lifeline: www.988lifeline.org
American Foundation for Suicide Prevention: www.afsp.org
American Psychiatric Association: www.psychiatry.org
Active Minds: www.activeminds.org
Clubhouse International: www.clubhouse-intl.org
Depression and Bipolar Support Alliance:
www.dbsalliance.org
Mental Health America: www.mhanational.org
National Alliance on Mental Illness: www.nami.org
National Council for Mental Wellbeing:
www.thenationalcouncil.org
National Institute of Mental Health: www.nimh.nih.gov
Schizophrenia & Psychosis Action Alliance:
www.sczaction.org
Substance Abuse and Mental Health Services Administration:
www.samhsa.gov

ACKNOWLEDGMENTS

Vince Granata dedicated an immense amount of time and energy to supporting this work. Over the course of three years, I gained more insight into creative writing and the publication process than I could have ever imagined. Not once did he ask for anything in return. From the very beginning, he believed in me, and I am eternally grateful for his expertise, guidance, and unwavering contributions.

I have great respect for Vince. If you haven't read his memoir *Everything Is Fine* yet, please do. His family's story is important, and can help us understand mental health from a loved one's perspective. His brother Tim, whom I have written letters to, deserves empathy and care. He is not a monster.

This memoir wouldn't be what it is without support from many of my family, friends, and colleagues.

My dear friend Katie Dipuma has been an incredible support throughout this journey. She took an active role, reading multiple versions of my manuscript and consistently offering thoughtful, constructive feedback. Katie was there for me when I struggled during and after graduate school. She helped me gain the courage to share my story. I am deeply grateful for our friendship and for our shared mission as social workers dedicated to helping those in need.

I am thankful to Todd French, whom I connected with for a peer perspective on my work. He went above and beyond, offering invaluable insight. It's been an honor to have had the opportunity to get to know him over the years.

To my girlfriend, Elizabeth Finger, a great person and social worker. Her care and support has been vital not only for my mental health but also in helping me share my story. From reading drafts to advocating for me and standing by me as I spoke to hundreds, I am stronger and better because she has been by my side.

To my friends Janice Bartleson, Jason Ehman, and Joe Storms, and my coworkers Deborah Faust, Glenn Liebman, Joan Dickinson, and Melissa Ramirez. Every one of them provided support at various points during my five years of writing this book. I've been incredibly fortunate to have had a team of knowledgeable and compassionate individuals supporting me throughout this process.

I am truly appreciative to my agent, Jeff Schmidt, for his tireless efforts in helping this book find a home. My heartfelt thanks go to everyone at Post Hill Press, including Caitlin Burdette, Debra Englander, and Sara Ann Alexander. I'm also thankful to Cynthia DelConte, whose exceptional work on my author portrait and cover photo brought this book to life.

Lastly, I want to recognize my family, including my parents and siblings, for the unwavering love and support they've shown me throughout my life. So many of them have been directly involved in this memoir—whether through read-throughs, thoughtful conversations, or helping me find answers to the questions that arose while I was writing. I wouldn't be who I am without each of them.

ABOUT THE AUTHOR

Cohen Miles-Rath is an author, speaker, advocate, and mental health professional. His work has supported mental health related policies such as workforce funding and education. He has facilitated over fifty training sessions, including Mental Health First Aid and Introduction to Trauma-Sensitive Schools. He has spoken to high school and college students, mental and behavioral health professionals, and elected officials, most notably Xavier Becerra, the US Secretary of Health and Human Services, at a 2023 Mental Health Round Table. He has shared his story and expertise for media including the *National Alliance of Mental Illness* blog and New York State Capitol press conferences. He holds a bachelor's in sociology and communications from SUNY Geneseo, and a master's degree in social work with a focus on community, policy, and political social action from Stony Brook University.

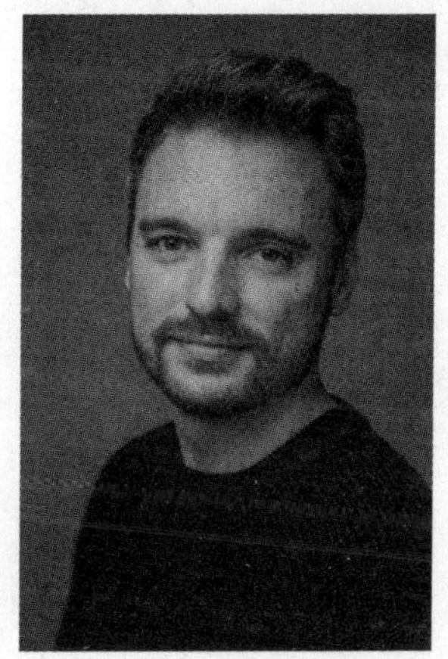

Delconte Photography LLC